MALE FERTILITY COOKBOOK

Healthy Recipes to Boost Male Fertility and Improve Sperm Quality.

Gabriela M. Whitehair

All rights reserved. No part of this publication may be reproduced, distributed, or transmitted in any form or by any means, including photocopying, recording, or other electronic or mechanical methods, without the prior written permission of the publisher, except in the case of brief quotations embodied in critical reviews and certain other noncommercial uses permitted by copyright law.

Copyright © Gabriela M. Whitehair, 2022.

TABLE OF CONTENT

INTRODUCTION

CHAPTER ONE
What is Male Fertility?

CHAPTER TWO
Male Fertility Factors

Lifestyle Choices That Impact Male Fertility

Nutrition and Male Fertility

CHAPTER THREE
Supplements and Male Fertility

Herbs and Male Fertility

Stress Management and Male Fertility

Exercise and Male Fertility

CHAPTER FOUR

Common Health Conditions and Male Fertility

Common Tests and Treatments for Male Fertility

Common Questions About Male Fertility

CHAPTER FIVE

MEAL PLAN

Day 1

Day 2

Day 3

Day 4

Day 5

Day 6

Day 7

CHAPTER SIX

FERTILITY RECIPES

BREAKFAST

LUNCH

DINNER

SNACK

DESSERT

SMOOTHIES

CONCLUSION

INTRODUCTION

Michael and his wife had been trying to have a baby for years but to no avail. After seeing multiple doctors, they were told that Michael had a lower-than-average sperm count and that their chances of conceiving were slim.

Not wanting to give up, Michael decided to take matters into his own hands and started researching ways to increase male fertility through nutrition.

He learned that certain vitamins and minerals, such as zinc and selenium, could play a role in increasing fertility. He also started to focus on eating more fresh fruits and vegetables, whole grains, and lean proteins.

He cut out processed foods, alcohol, and caffeine, and started getting better sleep.

Within a few months, Michael began to see a real difference. His sperm count had increased significantly, and his overall energy levels were higher. He and his wife were elated.

A few months later, Michael and his wife were delighted to discover that they were expecting a baby. After years of trying, they finally achieved their dream.

Michael was grateful that he had taken the time to research and implement a diet that had improved his fertility. He was now a proud father-to-be, and he was looking forward to the future with his growing family.

Male fertility refers to the ability of a male to father a child. It is determined by the quality and quantity of sperm that a man produces.

Male fertility can be affected by a variety of factors, such as age, lifestyle, diet, and health. To maximize fertility, it is important to make healthy lifestyle choices and seek medical advice if needed.

There are also several treatments and therapies available to improve male fertility.

By understanding male fertility and the factors that can affect it, couples can take steps to improve their chances of conceiving.

CHAPTER ONE

What is Male Fertility?

Male fertility refers to the ability of a man to impregnate a female partner. It involves a complex process involving the production of healthy sperm, its transportation to the female reproductive tract, and its ability to fertilize an egg.

It is well known that fertility declines with age, particularly for men. This is due to a decrease in the quality and quantity of sperm produced. The decline in fertility starts in the late 30s, with a more significant decrease after the age of 40. Other factors such as smoking, excessive alcohol consumption, obesity, and certain medications can also affect fertility.

There are several tests available to measure male fertility. These include a semen analysis which evaluates the number, shape, and motility of sperm, as well as a hormone test to determine levels of testosterone and other hormones.

Additionally, a scrotal ultrasound can be used to detect any blockages or abnormalities in the sperm ducts.

If a man is having difficulty getting his partner pregnant, there are treatment options available. These include lifestyle changes such as quitting smoking, eating a healthy diet, and exercising regularly.

Also, a doctor may recommend medications or fertility treatments such as intrauterine insemination (IUI) or in vitro fertilization (IVF).

It is important to remember that male infertility is not an indicator of masculinity or a lack of virility. It is a medical condition that can be treated and managed.

CHAPTER TWO

Male Fertility Factors

Male fertility is an important factor when it comes to conception and successful pregnancy. If a man is infertile, it can be difficult for a couple to conceive a baby naturally.

A man's fertility is affected by many factors, including age, lifestyle, health, and genetic factors.

Age is a major factor in male fertility. As a man gets older, his sperm production decreases, and the quality of his sperm may also decrease. This is why it is important for men to stay as healthy as possible and take steps to protect their fertility.

Lifestyle factors can also affect male fertility. Smoking, drinking alcohol, using illegal drugs, and exposure to environmental toxins can all damage sperm and reduce fertility.

Stress can also have an effect, so it is important to manage stress levels and maintain a healthy lifestyle.

Health issues can also affect male fertility. Certain health conditions, such as diabetes and obesity, can interfere with sperm production. Other conditions, such as an undescended testicle or a varicocele (an enlarged vein in the scrotum) can also reduce fertility.

Finally, genetics can affect male fertility. Some genetic conditions, such as cystic fibrosis, can reduce fertility. Other conditions, such as Klinefelter syndrome, can cause a man to have no sperm at all.

Male fertility can be improved by making lifestyle changes, such as quitting smoking and reducing alcohol consumption.

Maintaining a healthy weight, eating a balanced diet, and reducing stress levels can also help. In some cases, medical interventions, such as assisted reproductive technology, may be required. Although male fertility is an important factor in conception, it is not the only factor.

Female fertility is also important, and couples should discuss their fertility options with a doctor.

With the right care, many couples can successfully conceive a baby. No matter what, it is important for men to take steps to protect their fertility. By making healthy lifestyle choices and seeing a doctor regularly, men can increase their chances of becoming a father.

Lifestyle Choices That Impact Male Fertility

Male fertility is a complex topic, and there are several choices that men can make that can have an effect on their fertility.

Some of these choices can be lifestyle related, such as smoking, drinking alcohol, or taking certain medications or supplements.

Other choices may be related to diet, such as eating a balanced diet, avoiding processed foods, and maintaining a healthy weight.

Smoking cigarettes has been linked to male infertility, as it can reduce sperm count and damage sperm. Additionally, men who are exposed to secondhand smoke may be at a higher risk for fertility issues.

It is recommended that men who wish to become fathers should avoid smoking in order to protect their fertility.

Drinking alcohol can also reduce fertility in men. Heavy drinking can reduce sperm production, as well as damage sperm.

Additionally, alcohol can increase levels of testosterone, which can make it more difficult for a man to become pregnant. It is recommended that men who are trying to conceive limit their alcohol consumption.

Certain medications and supplements have also been linked to male infertility. Men should be careful when taking these medications and should discuss any concerns with their doctor.

Additionally, men should be aware of any side effects that could potentially reduce fertility.

Men should also pay attention to their diet. Eating a balanced diet can help protect a man's fertility.

Eating a variety of fruits and vegetables, whole grains, and lean proteins can help maintain a healthy weight and protect fertility.

Additionally, avoiding processed foods and foods high in saturated fats can help protect fertility.

Finally, men should be aware of the impact of environmental toxins. Exposure to certain toxins, such as pesticides and herbicides, can reduce fertility in men.

It is recommended that men avoid contact with these toxins to protect their fertility.

Overall, there are many choices that men can make that can impact their fertility. By making informed decisions about lifestyle, diet, medications, and environmental exposure.

Nutrition and Male Fertility

Nutrition plays an important role in male fertility. A balanced diet is necessary for proper reproductive health and optimal sperm production.

Adequate intake of essential nutrients, such as protein, carbohydrates, fats, vitamins, and minerals, is necessary for proper sperm production and healthy sperm function.

Macronutrients, such as carbohydrates, proteins, and fats, are needed to provide the energy necessary for sperm production and maturation, while micronutrients, such as vitamins and minerals, are essential for proper sperm development.

Foods that are rich in antioxidants, such as fruits and vegetables, may help to protect sperm from damage caused by free radicals.

Additionally, foods that are rich in omega-3 fatty acids, such as fish, nuts, and seeds, may help to improve sperm quality.

Inadequate intake of essential nutrients, such as zinc and folate, has been linked to decreased sperm count and motility, as well as increased DNA damage in sperm.

Zinc is especially important for healthy sperm production, as it helps to support the production of testosterone, which is essential for sperm maturation.

Additionally, folate is important for sperm health, as it helps to protect genetic material contained in sperm from damage.

Overall, maintaining a balanced diet that is rich in essential nutrients is important for male fertility.

Eating a variety of nutrient-dense foods, such as fruits, vegetables, lean proteins, whole grains, nuts, and seeds, can help to support healthy sperm production and function.

Additionally, avoiding processed and refined foods, as well as limiting alcohol and caffeine intake, may help to optimize male fertility.

CHAPTER THREE

Supplements and Male Fertility

Supplements are a great way to improve male fertility. Studies have shown that men who take certain supplements can experience an improved sperm count, motility, and morphology, which can all lead to improved fertility.

Some of the most common supplements used to improve male fertility are zinc, folic acid, omega-3 fatty acids, and vitamins C and E.

Zinc is a mineral that plays an important role in many bodily functions, including male fertility.

Zinc helps to keep sperm healthy and active, and studies have found that men taking zinc supplements have higher sperm counts.

Folic acid is also important for male fertility. Folic acid helps with sperm production and motility, as well as protecting DNA from damage, which can lead to improved sperm quality and fertility.

Omega-3 fatty acids are also beneficial for male fertility, as they help to improve blood flow to the testicles, which can improve sperm production. Vitamins C and E are also important for male fertility, as they help to reduce inflammation and oxidative stress, which can have a negative effect on sperm production.

Herbs and Male Fertility

Herbs have been used for centuries to help men improve their fertility. Herbal remedies are becoming increasingly popular for male fertility as they are less expensive than other treatments and generally have fewer side effects.

Ginseng is one of the most popular herbs for male fertility. It has been shown to improve sperm quality, increase testosterone levels, and improve erectile function. It is also known to reduce stress levels, which can help improve fertility.

Maca root is another popular herb for male fertility. This herb has been found to increase sperm count and motility, as well as improve libido. Maca root is also known to increase fertility in men suffering from low testosterone levels.

Tribulus terrestris is an herb that has been used in traditional medicine for many years. It has been found to improve sperm count, motility, and morphology, as well as improve libido.

Ginkgo biloba is a herb that has been used in traditional medicine for centuries. It is known to improve sperm quality, increase testosterone levels, and improve blood flow to the genitals. Ginkgo biloba is also known to reduce stress levels and improve fertility.

Saw palmetto is an herb that has been found to improve sperm count, motility, and morphology. It is also known to reduce DHT levels, which can help improve fertility.

These are just a few of the many herbs that can be used to improve male fertility. While herbs may not be a miracle cure, they can be an effective way to naturally improve fertility.

Stress Management and Male Fertility

Stress management is essential for male fertility. Stress can have a detrimental effect on the body, and this is especially true when it comes to male fertility.

Stress can lead to a disruption in menstrual cycles, erectile dysfunction, and a decrease in overall sperm production and quality. All of these factors can have a negative impact on a man's ability to conceive.

There are several ways to manage stress and improve male fertility. Exercise is an excellent way to reduce stress, as it releases endorphins that act as a natural mood booster. Additionally, participating in activities like yoga and meditation can help to reduce stress and improve overall health.

Additionally, getting enough sleep is important for stress management, as sleep deprivation can increase levels of stress hormones in the body.

It's important to talk to a doctor about any stress-related issues, as certain medications and treatments can help to reduce stress and improve fertility.

Stress management is an important part of improving male fertility. Participating in activities like exercise, yoga, and meditation, getting enough sleep, eating a balanced diet, and speaking to a doctor can all help to reduce stress and improve male fertility.

Exercise and Male Fertility

Exercise has been found to have a positive effect on male fertility. Regular exercise can help reduce stress and improve overall health, both of which can play an important role in male fertility.

Exercise can help to improve the quality of semen, such as increasing the sperm count, motility, and morphology. It can also help to reduce testosterone levels which can improve sperm production. Additionally, exercise can help to increase circulation which can improve blood flow to the testicles and support healthy sperm production.

Exercise can also help to reduce body fat which can have a positive effect on male fertility. Lower levels of body fat can help to improve hormone production and reduce the risk of conditions such as obesity, which can have a negative effect on fertility.

Finally, exercise can help to reduce levels of oxidative stress which can damage sperm DNA. Exercise has been found to reduce levels of oxidative stress, which can help to improve sperm quality.

Exercises can have a positive impact on male fertility. It can help to improve the quality of semen, reduce body fat, and reduce oxidative stress. Therefore, it is important for men to get regular physical activity to support their fertility.

It can also help to reduce stress which can help to improve mental health and reduce the risk of conditions such as depression, which can have a negative effect on fertility.

CHAPTER FOUR

Common Health Conditions and Male Fertility

There are several health conditions that can affect male fertility, some of which are treatable and some that are not.

One of the most common health conditions that can affect male fertility is low sperm count. Low sperm count is usually a result of hormonal imbalances or poor sperm production.

Treatment for this condition may include lifestyle changes, medication, or fertility treatments.

Medications such as clomiphene citrate and human chorionic gonadotropin (hCG) can help to increase sperm count.

Fertility treatments such as in vitro fertilization (IVF) or intracytoplasmic sperm injection (ICSI) may also be used to improve sperm quality and quantity.

Another health condition that can affect male fertility is erectile dysfunction (ED). ED is a condition in which a man is unable to get or maintain an erection. This condition is often caused by psychological factors such as stress, anxiety, or depression and can also be caused by physical factors such as diabetes, obesity, or heart disease. Treatment for ED may include lifestyle changes, medication, or therapy.

Varicocele is another common health condition that can affect male fertility. Varicocele is a condition in which the veins in the scrotum become enlarged, resulting in poor sperm production. Treatment for this condition usually involves surgery to repair the veins.

Finally, genetic disorders can also affect male fertility. Genetic disorders such as Klinefelter Syndrome, cystic fibrosis, and hemophilia can all have an effect on fertility.

Treatment for these conditions may involve lifestyle changes, medication, or genetic counseling.

Common Tests and Treatments for Male Fertility

Male fertility tests are used to determine the cause of infertility and to assess the reproductive health of a man. Common tests for male fertility include semen analysis, endocrine testing, and genetic testing.

- Semen Analysis: A semen analysis is the most common male fertility test. It examines the quality, quantity, and maturity of sperm in a man's semen sample. It can determine the percentage of motile (swimming) sperm, as well as the overall number of sperm present.

Results of a semen analysis can help identify abnormalities such as low sperm count, poor sperm motility, or abnormal sperm morphology.

- Endocrine Testing: Endocrine testing examines the levels of various hormones in a man's blood. These hormones, such as follicle-stimulating hormone (FSH) and testosterone, play an important role in fertility and sexual health.

Abnormal results can indicate a variety of conditions, including hypogonadism and polycystic ovary syndrome.

- Genetic Testing: Genetic testing can help identify any genetic abnormalities that may be impacting a man's fertility. These tests can detect chromosomal abnormalities, gene mutations, and other genetic disorders that can cause infertility.

These tests are important for helping to diagnose the cause of infertility and to determine the best treatment options.

There are a variety of treatments available for male infertility, depending on the underlying cause.

- Hormonal Treatment: Hormonal

treatments are often the first line of treatment for male infertility. This involves prescribing medications to correct any hormonal imbalances that may be contributing to infertility.

These medications may include testosterone, human chorionic gonadotropin (hCG), and clomiphene citrate.

- Surgery: Surgery may be

recommended in some cases of male infertility. This may involve repairing any physical abnormalities, such as varicoceles, or removing any blockages in the male reproductive tract.

- Assisted Reproductive Technology (ART): ART is a type of fertility treatment that involves the use of laboratory techniques to assist with conception. This may include in vitro fertilization (IVF), intracytoplasmic sperm injection (ICSI), and donor insemination.

- Lifestyle Changes: In some cases, male infertility can be treated with lifestyle changes. This may involve stopping smoking, avoiding recreational drugs, and reducing alcohol consumption.

Maintaining a healthy weight and exercising regularly can also help to improve fertility.

- Supplements: Certain supplements

may also be helpful in improving fertility. These may include vitamins and minerals, such as zinc and folic acid, as well as herbs, such as ginseng and maca root.

In some cases, no treatment may be necessary. This is usually the case when the cause of male infertility is unknown or when the male partner has a low sperm count but the sperm is of good quality.

In such cases, couples may be advised to try natural conception methods.

Overall, male infertility is a complex condition and the treatment will depend on the underlying cause.

Common Questions About Male Fertility

1. Does diet affect male fertility?

Yes, diet can have an effect on male fertility. Eating a healthy diet with plenty of fruits, vegetables, and whole grains, as well as avoiding processed and high-sugar foods, can help improve fertility.

Getting enough essential vitamins and minerals from food sources can help promote fertility.

2. Does age affect male fertility?

Yes, age can have an effect on male fertility. As men age, sperm production may decline, making it more difficult to conceive.

Age-related health conditions such as diabetes, obesity, and high blood pressure can also have a negative impact on male fertility.

3. Does smoking affect male fertility?

Yes, smoking can have a negative effect on male fertility. Smoking can reduce sperm count and lower sperm quality, making it more difficult to conceive.

Smoking can increase the risk of erectile dysfunction, which can also reduce fertility.

4. Does alcohol affect male fertility?

Yes, alcohol can have an effect on male fertility. Heavy drinking can reduce sperm quality and decrease sperm count, making it more difficult to conceive.

Alcohol can also increase the risk of erectile dysfunction, which can also reduce fertility.

5. Does stress affect male fertility?

Yes, stress can have an effect on male fertility. Stress can cause a decrease in sperm count, as well as reduce the quality of sperm.

Additionally, stress can lead to erectile dysfunction, which can further reduce fertility.

6. Does medication affect male fertility?

Yes, certain medications can have an effect on male fertility. Certain medications, such as chemotherapy and radiation therapy, can cause a decrease in sperm count and quality.

Additionally, some medications used to treat chronic health conditions can also have a negative effect on fertility.

7. Does obesity affect male fertility?

Yes, obesity can have an effect on male fertility. Being overweight can cause a decrease in sperm count and quality, making it more difficult to conceive.

Additionally, obesity can increase the risk of erectile dysfunction, which can further reduce fertility.

8. Does exercise affect male fertility?

Yes, exercise can have an effect on male fertility. Exercising regularly can help improve fertility by promoting a healthy weight, reducing stress, and improving overall health.

Exercises can also improve blood circulation, which can also help improve fertility.

9. Does environmental exposure affect male fertility?

Yes, environmental exposure can have an effect on male fertility. Exposure to certain chemicals, such as pesticides and industrial pollutants, can reduce sperm count and quality, making it more difficult to conceive.

Additionally, exposure to radiation can also have a negative effect on fertility.

10. Does chronic illness affect male fertility?
Yes, chronic illnesses can have an effect on male fertility. Certain chronic illnesses, such as diabetes and high blood pressure, can cause a decrease in sperm count and quality, making it more difficult to conceive.

Chronic illnesses can also increase the risk of erectile dysfunction, which can further reduce fertility.

11. Does sexually transmitted infection affect male fertility?

Yes, sexually transmitted infections (STIs) can have an effect on male fertility. Certain STIs, such as chlamydia and gonorrhea, can cause a decrease in sperm count and quality, making it more difficult to conceive.

STIs can also increase the risk of erectile dysfunction, which can further reduce fertility.

12. Does tight underwear affect male fertility?

Yes, tight underwear can have an effect on male fertility. Tight underwear can cause an increase in temperature in the testicles, which can reduce sperm count and quality, making it more difficult to conceive.

CHAPTER FIVE

MEAL PLAN

Day 1:

Breakfast: Overnight oats with chia seeds, walnuts, and blueberries

Ingredients:
- 1/2 cup rolled oats
- 2 tablespoons chia seeds
- 1/2 cup almond milk
- 1/2 teaspoon vanilla extract
- 1/4 teaspoon ground cinnamon
- 1/4 cup walnuts, chopped
- 1/4 cup blueberries

Instructions:

1. In a medium bowl, combine the oats, chia seeds, almond milk, vanilla extract, and cinnamon. Stir until all ingredients are well combined.

2. Cover the bowl and place in the refrigerator overnight.

3. The next morning, remove the bowl from the refrigerator and stir in the walnuts and blueberries.

4. Divide the mixture into two bowls and enjoy.

Prep Time: 10 minutes
Chill Time: 8 hours

Lunch: Quinoa salad with avocado, cherry tomatoes, and grilled chicken

Ingredients:
- 2 cups cooked quinoa
- 1/2 avocado, cubed
- 1/2 cup cherry tomatoes, halved
- 2 grilled chicken breasts, diced
- 2 tablespoons olive oil
- 2 tablespoons lime juice
- 1/4 teaspoon garlic powder
- Salt and pepper, to taste

Instructions:
1. Cook the quinoa according to package instructions. Set aside and let cool.

2. In a large bowl, combine the cooled quinoa, avocado, cherry tomatoes, and grilled chicken.

3. In a small bowl, whisk together the olive oil, lime juice, garlic powder, salt, and pepper.

4. Pour the dressing over the quinoa mixture and gently toss to combine.

5. Serve the quinoa salad immediately or chill for up to 2 days.

Prep Time: 15 minutes

Snack: Smoothie with banana, almond milk, and spinach

Ingredients:

-1 banana

-1/2 cup almond milk

-1/2 cup spinach

Instructions:

1. Peel and cut the banana into small slices.

2. Put the banana slices into a blender.

3. Add the almond milk and spinach.

4. Blend the ingredients until the mixture is thick and smooth.

Prep Time: 5 minutes

Dinner: Baked salmon with roasted vegetables and quinoa

Ingredients:

- 4 salmon fillets
- 2 tablespoons olive oil
- Salt and pepper to taste
- 2 red bell peppers, cut into 1-inch cubes
- 1 red onion, cut into 1-inch cubes
- 1 zucchini, cut into 1-inch cubes
- 1 pint cherry tomatoes
- 2 cloves garlic, minced
- 2 tablespoons fresh parsley, chopped
- 1 cup quinoa
- 2 cups vegetable broth

Instructions:

Preparation Time: 10 minutes

Cook Time: 40 minutes

1. Preheat the oven to 400°F.

2. Place salmon fillets on a baking sheet and brush with olive oil. Season with salt and pepper.

3. Place bell peppers, onion, zucchini, and cherry tomatoes on a separate baking sheet. Drizzle with olive oil, season with salt and pepper, and toss to coat.

4. Place both baking sheets in the preheated oven and bake for 20 minutes.

5. Meanwhile, prepare the quinoa according to package instructions.

6. After 20 minutes, add the garlic to the vegetables and cook for an additional 10 minutes.

7. When everything is done cooking, remove from the oven and assemble. Place the quinoa on a plate, top with the vegetables and salmon, and sprinkle with parsley. Enjoy!

Day 2:

Breakfast: Greek yogurt with hemp seeds, walnuts, and honey

Ingredients:
- 2 cups Greek yogurt
- 2 tablespoons hemp seeds

- 2 tablespoons walnuts, chopped

- 2 tablespoons honey

Instructions:

1. In a medium bowl, combine the Greek yogurt, hemp seeds, walnuts, and honey.

2. Mix together until all ingredients are evenly combined.

3. Serve the yogurt mixture in a bowl and enjoy!

Prep Time: 5 minutes

Lunch: Lentil soup with spinach and kale

Ingredients:

- 2 tablespoons olive oil
- 1 onion, diced
- 2 cloves garlic, minced
- 1 teaspoon ground cumin
- 1 teaspoon ground coriander
- 4 cups vegetable broth
- 2 cups dried lentils
- 1 can diced tomatoes
- 2 cups baby spinach
- 2 cups kale, chopped
- Salt and pepper to taste

Instructions:

1. Heat the olive oil in a large pot over medium heat.

2. Add the onion and garlic and sauté until the onion is softened, about 2 minutes.

3. Add the cumin and coriander and cook for an additional minute.

4. Pour in the vegetable broth and lentils and bring to a boil.

5. Reduce the heat to low and simmer for 20 minutes, or until the lentils are tender.

6. Stir in the diced tomatoes, spinach and kale and cook for an additional 5 minutes.

7. Season with salt and pepper to taste.

8. Serve warm.

Prep Time: 10 minutes

Cook Time: 25 minutes

Snack: Apple slices with almond butter

Ingredients:

- 2 Apples

- 2 tablespoons of Almond butter
- 2 teaspoons of Honey
- 4 tablespoons of Sliced Almonds

Instructions:

1. Preheat the oven to 350°F.

2. Cut apples into thin slices and place them on a baking sheet.

3. Spread almond butter and honey over the apple slices.

4. Sprinkle with sliced almonds.

5. Bake for 10-15 minutes, or until the edges of the apples are golden brown.

6. Serve and enjoy!

Prep Time: 10 minutes
Cook Time: 15 minutes

Dinner: Stir-fry vegetables with brown rice and tofu

Ingredients
- 2 tbsp of sesame oil
- 2 cloves of garlic, minced
- 5 cups of mixed vegetables (such as broccoli, carrots, bell peppers, snow peas, mushrooms, etc.)
- 1/2 block of extra-firm tofu, cubed
- 1/4 cup of tamari (soy sauce)
- 2 cups of cooked brown rice
- Sesame seeds and green onions for garnish

Instructions

1. Heat the sesame oil in a large wok or skillet over medium-high heat.

2. Add the minced garlic and stir-fry for 30 seconds.

3. Add the vegetables and tofu and stir-fry for 4 minutes, or until the vegetables are just tender.

4. Add the tamari and stir-fry for an additional minute.

5. Add the cooked brown rice and stir-fry for 2 minutes, or until everything is heated through.

6. Garnish with sesame seeds and green onions, if desired.

7. Serve warm.

Prep Time: 10 minutes
Cook Time: 10 minutes
Total Time: 20 minutes

Day 3:

Breakfast: Scrambled eggs with mushrooms, bell peppers, and spinach

Ingredients:
- 2 large eggs
- 2 tablespoons of butter

- 1/2 cup of mushrooms, diced
- 1/2 cup of bell peppers, diced
- Salt and pepper to taste

Instructions:

1. Gather together all the ingredients.

2. Heat a skillet over medium heat and add butter.

3. Once butter is melted, add mushrooms and bell peppers to the skillet and cook until softened, about 5 minutes.

4. Crack the eggs into a bowl, add salt and pepper, and whisk together until combined.

5. Add egg mixture to the skillet and scramble until eggs are cooked through, about 5 minutes.

6. Serve immediately.

Prep Time: 10 minutes
Lunch: Kale salad with roasted sweet potatoes, mango, and avocado

Ingredients:
- 2 medium sweet potatoes, peeled and diced
- 2 tablespoons olive oil
- 2 bunches of kale, washed and chopped
- 2 tablespoons honey
- 2 tablespoons balsamic vinegar
- Salt and pepper to taste
- 1 mango, peeled and diced

- 1 avocado, peeled and diced

Instructions:

1. Preheat the oven to 425 degrees Fahrenheit.

2. Place diced sweet potatoes on a baking sheet and toss with olive oil, salt, and pepper.

3. Bake for 20-25 minutes or until the sweet potatoes are lightly browned.

4. In a large bowl, combine kale, honey, and balsamic vinegar.

5. Massage the dressing into the kale until it's lightly coated.

6. Add the roasted sweet potatoes, mango, and avocado to the bowl and toss.

7. Serve the salad immediately.

Prep Time: 10 minutes
Cook Time: 25 minutes
Total Time: 35 minutes

Snack: Carrot sticks with hummus

Ingredients:
-4-5 large carrots
-1/4 cup hummus
-1/8 teaspoon garlic powder
-1/4 teaspoon of fresh ground black pepper

Instructions:

1. Preheat the oven to 375 degrees.

2. Peel and cut the carrots into thin sticks.

3. Place the carrots on a baking sheet and sprinkle with garlic powder and black pepper.

4. Bake the carrots in the preheated oven for 15-20 minutes or until they are tender.

5. Remove the carrots from the oven and let them cool.

6. Serve the carrot sticks with hummus.

Prep Time: 10 minutes

Cook Time: 20 minutes
Total Time: 30 minutes

Dinner: Baked cod with quinoa and roasted Brussels sprouts

Ingredients:
- 4 (4-ounce) cod fillets
- 1/2 teaspoon ground black pepper
- 1/4 teaspoon salt
- 2 tablespoons olive oil
- 1 cup quinoa
- 2 cups chicken broth
- 1/2 teaspoon garlic powder
- 1/2 teaspoon dried oregano
- 1/2 teaspoon dried thyme
- 1/4 teaspoon paprika
- 1/4 teaspoon ground cumin

- 1 pound Brussels sprouts, halved
- 2 tablespoons olive oil
- 2 cloves garlic, minced

Instructions:
- Preheat the oven to 400 degrees F.

- Season cod fillets with pepper and salt. Heat 2 tablespoons of olive oil in a large oven-safe skillet over medium-high heat. Add cod to skillet and cook until golden brown, about 3 minutes per side. Transfer to a plate and set aside.

- In the same skillet, add quinoa, chicken broth, garlic powder, oregano, thyme, paprika, and cumin. Bring to a boil, reduce heat to low and simmer for 15 minutes.

- Meanwhile, place Brussels sprouts on a baking sheet and toss with remaining 2 tablespoons of olive oil, minced garlic, and salt and pepper to taste. Roast for 15 minutes.

- Place cod on top of quinoa and bake for 10 minutes, or until cod is cooked through.

- Serve cod with quinoa and Brussels sprouts.

Prep Time: 15 minutes
Cook Time: 30 minutes

Day 4:

Breakfast: Oatmeal with almond milk, banana, and flaxseeds

Ingredients:
- ¾ cup of old-fashioned rolled oats
- 2 cups of almond milk
- 1 banana, sliced
- 1 tablespoon of flaxseeds

Instructions:
1. In a medium saucepan, bring 2 cups of almond milk to a gentle boil.

2. Add the rolled oats and reduce the heat to low.

3. Cook for 5 minutes, stirring occasionally, until the oats are softened.

4. Add the banana slices and flaxseeds and cook for an additional 2 minutes.

5. Serve the oatmeal warm and enjoy!

Prep Time: 10 minutes

Lunch: Quinoa bowl with black beans, corn, and tomato

Ingredients:
-1 cup quinoa
-1 can black beans, rinsed and drained
-1 cup corn
-1 cup diced tomatoes, fresh or canned
-2 tablespoons olive oil
-2 cloves garlic, minced

-1 teaspoon chili powder

-1/2 teaspoon ground cumin

-Salt and pepper to taste

Instructions:

1. Cook quinoa according to package instructions.

2. Heat olive oil in a large skillet over medium heat. Add garlic and sauté for 1-2 minutes.

3. Add black beans, corn, tomatoes, chili powder, cumin, and salt and pepper. Cook for 5-7 minutes, stirring occasionally.

4. Add cooked quinoa to the skillet and stir to combine. Cook for an additional 3-5 minutes.

5. Serve quinoa bowl warm and enjoy!

Prep Time: 10 minutes
Cook Time: 15 minutes

Snack: Smoothie with banana, almond milk, and spinach

Ingredients:
- 1 banana
- 2 cups of spinach
- 2 cups of almond milk

Prep time: 5 minutes

Instructions:

1. Peel and slice the banana into small chunks.

2. Place the banana chunks and spinach into a blender.

3. Pour the almond milk over the banana and spinach.

4. Blend until the smoothie is at the desired consistency.

5. Serve the smoothie and enjoy!

Dinner: Grilled chicken with roasted vegetables and brown rice

Ingredients:
- 4 boneless and skinless chicken breasts
- 2 tablespoons of olive oil
- 1 teaspoon of garlic powder
- 1 teaspoon of dried oregano
- 1 teaspoon of paprika
- 1/2 teaspoon of black pepper
- 1/2 teaspoon of salt
- 2 zucchini, sliced
- 2 bell peppers, diced
- 1 red onion, sliced
- 1 cup of brown rice
- 2 tablespoons of butter
- 2 cups of water

Instructions:

1. Preheat the grill to medium heat.

2. In a small bowl, whisk together olive oil, garlic powder, oregano, paprika, black pepper and salt.

3. Brush the chicken breasts with the olive oil mixture.

4. Place the chicken breasts on the preheated grill. Cook for 8-10 minutes, flipping the chicken halfway through, or until chicken is cooked through.

5. In a medium bowl, toss the zucchini, bell peppers and red onion with a tablespoon of olive oil and a pinch of salt and pepper.

6. Place the vegetables onto the grill and cook for 8-10 minutes, flipping halfway through.

7. Meanwhile, bring the butter and water to a boil in a medium pot. Add the brown rice, reduce the heat to low, cover and cook for 30 minutes or until all the water is absorbed.

8. Serve the grilled chicken with roasted vegetables and brown rice.

Prep time: 10 minutes
Cook time: 50 minutes

Day 5:

Breakfast: Chia pudding with almond milk, blueberries, and walnuts

Ingredients:
- 1/2 cup chia seeds
- 2 cups almond milk
- 1/3 cup fresh blueberries
- 1/4 cup chopped walnuts
- 2 tablespoons honey
- 1/4 teaspoon ground cinnamon

Instructions:

1. In a medium bowl, combine chia seeds and almond milk. Stir to combine.

2. Cover the bowl and let sit in the refrigerator overnight.

3. In the morning, stir the chia pudding and add honey and cinnamon. Stir to combine.

4. Divide the pudding into two bowls.

5. Top each bowl with half of the blueberries and walnuts.

6. Serve and enjoy!

Prep Time: 10 minutes
Chill Time: 8 hours

Lunch: Lentil soup with spinach and kale

Ingredients:
- 1 cup of green lentils
- 2 cloves of garlic, minced

- 2 tablespoons of olive oil
- 2 carrots, peeled and diced
- 1 onion, diced
- 2 stalks of celery, diced
- 4 cups of vegetable broth
- 1 teaspoon of dried thyme
- 1/2 teaspoon of ground cumin
- 1/2 teaspoon of ground coriander
- 1/4 teaspoon of cayenne pepper
- 2 cups of chopped kale
- 2 cups of chopped spinach
- Salt and pepper to taste

Instructions:

1. Heat the olive oil in a large pot over medium heat.

2. Add the garlic, carrots, onion, and celery and sauté for 5 minutes.

3. Add the lentils, vegetable broth, thyme, cumin, coriander, and cayenne pepper and bring to a boil.

4. Reduce the heat to low and simmer for 25 minutes, or until the lentils are tender.

5. Add the kale and spinach and simmer for 5 minutes.

6. Season with salt and pepper to taste.

7. Serve hot.

Prep Time: 10 minutes

Cook Time: 30 minutes

Snack: Apple slices with almond butter

Ingredients:
- 2 Apples (any type)
- 2 tablespoons Almond Butter
- 1 teaspoon Cinnamon
- 1 tablespoon Honey

Instructions:
1. Slice the apples into thin wedges.
2. Place the apple slices onto a plate.
3. Spread the almond butter evenly over the top of the apple slices.
4. Sprinkle the cinnamon over the top of the almond butter.
5. Drizzle the honey over the top.

6. Serve and enjoy!

Prep Time: 5 minutes

Dinner: Baked salmon with roasted vegetables and quinoa

Ingredients:
- 2 Salmon fillets
- 2 tablespoons olive oil
- Salt and pepper, to taste
- 1/2 cup uncooked quinoa
- 1 cup water
- 1/2 cup chopped bell peppers
- 1/2 cup chopped zucchini
- 1/2 cup chopped yellow squash
- 1/2 cup chopped mushrooms
- 1/4 cup chopped red onion

- 2 cloves garlic, minced
- 2 tablespoons chopped fresh parsley

Instructions:

1. Preheat the oven to 375°F.

2. Place salmon fillets in a baking dish. Drizzle with olive oil and season with salt and pepper.

3. Bake for 15-20 minutes, or until salmon is cooked through.

4. Meanwhile, combine quinoa and water in a medium saucepan. Bring to a boil, reduce heat to low and simmer for 15 minutes.

5. Meanwhile, in a large skillet, heat remaining olive oil over medium-high heat.

Add bell peppers, zucchini, yellow squash, mushrooms, red onion, and garlic. Cook until vegetables are tender, about 10 minutes.

6. Fluff quinoa with a fork and add to the skillet with the vegetables. Stir in parsley.

7. Serve the roasted vegetables and quinoa with the baked salmon.

Prep time: 25 minutes
Cook time: 20 minutes

Day 6:

Breakfast: Greek yogurt with hemp seeds, walnuts, and honey

Ingredients:
- 2 cups of plain Greek yogurt
- 2 tablespoons of hemp seeds
- 2 tablespoons of walnuts, chopped
- 2 tablespoons of honey

Instructions:
1. In a medium bowl, combine the Greek yogurt, hemp seeds, walnuts, and honey.

2. Mix until all the ingredients are evenly distributed.

3. Serve immediately.

Prep time: 5 minutes

Lunch: Kale salad with roasted sweet potatoes, mango, and avocado

Ingredients:
- 4 cups kale, chopped
- 2 sweet potatoes, peeled and diced
- 2 tablespoons olive oil
- 1 teaspoon salt
- ½ teaspoon black pepper
- 1 mango, peeled and diced
- 1 avocado, peeled and diced
- 2 tablespoons lemon juice
- ¼ cup feta cheese, crumbled (optional)

Instructions:

1. Preheat the oven to 350°F.

2. Place diced sweet potatoes on a baking sheet and drizzle with olive oil. Sprinkle it with salt and pepper.

3. Bake for 25-30 minutes, or until sweet potatoes are tender.

4. In a large bowl, combine kale, roasted sweet potatoes, mango, and avocado.

5. Drizzle with lemon juice and toss to combine.

6. Sprinkle with feta cheese, if using.

7. Serve and enjoy!

Prep Time: 10 minutes
Cook Time: 25-30 minutes
Total Time: 35-40 minutes

Snack: Carrot sticks with hummus

Ingredients:
- 4 large carrots, cut into sticks
- 2 tablespoons olive oil
- 1/4 teaspoon garlic powder
- 1/4 teaspoon onion powder
- 1/4 teaspoon smoked paprika
- Salt and pepper, to taste
- 1 (14-ounce) can chickpeas, drained and rinsed
- 2 tablespoons freshly squeezed lemon juice

- 2 tablespoons tahini
- 2 cloves garlic, minced
- 2 tablespoons olive oil
- 2-3 tablespoons water

Instructions:

1. Preheat the oven to 425°F. Line a baking sheet with parchment paper.

2. Place the carrot sticks in a bowl and add the olive oil, garlic powder, onion powder, smoked paprika, and salt and pepper, to taste. Toss to combine and spread evenly onto the prepared baking sheet.

3. Bake for 15-20 minutes, flipping the carrots halfway through.

4. Meanwhile, add the chickpeas, lemon juice, tahini, garlic, olive oil, and 2 tablespoons of water to a food processor. Pulse until smooth. If needed, add additional water until desired consistency is reached.

5. Serve the carrot sticks with the hummus.

Prep Time: 10 minutes
Cook Time: 20 minutes

Dinner: Stir-fry vegetables with brown rice and tofu

Ingredients:
- 3 cups vegetable broth
- 2 tablespoons soy sauce

- 2 tablespoons sesame oil
- 2 tablespoons rice vinegar
- 1 tablespoon honey
- 2 cloves garlic, minced
- 1 teaspoon freshly grated ginger
- 1 red bell pepper, sliced
- 1 cup sliced mushrooms
- 1 cup diced carrots
- 1 cup snow peas
- 1 cup diced tofu
- 2 cups cooked brown rice
- 2 tablespoons chopped fresh cilantro

Instructions:

1. In a large pot, bring the vegetable broth to a boil over medium-high heat.

2. Add the soy sauce, sesame oil, rice vinegar, honey, garlic, and ginger and stir to combine.

3. Add the bell pepper, mushrooms, carrots, and snow peas and reduce the heat to medium. Cook for 5 minutes.

4. Add the tofu and cook for an additional 5 minutes.

5. Add the cooked brown rice and stir to combine.

6. Sprinkle with cilantro and serve.

Prep Time: 10 minutes
Cook Time: 10 minutes

Day 7:

Breakfast: Scrambled eggs with mushrooms, bell peppers, and spinach

Ingredients:
- 2 eggs
- 2 tablespoons butter
- 2 tablespoons milk
- 1/4 cup of thinly sliced mushrooms
- 1/4 cup of diced bell peppers
- 1/4 cup of spinach

Instructions:

1. In a medium bowl, whisk together eggs, milk, and a pinch of salt and pepper.

2. Heat a large non-stick skillet over medium heat with the butter.

3. Add the mushrooms, bell peppers, and spinach to the skillet and cook until vegetables are tender, about 5 minutes.

4. Pour in the egg mixture and stir frequently with a rubber spatula, scraping the bottom of the pan until the eggs are set, about 5 minutes.

5. Serve the scrambled eggs with mushrooms, bell peppers, and spinach.

Prep Time: 10 minutes

Lunch: Quinoa bowl with black beans, corn, and tomato

Ingredients:

-1 cup quinoa

-1/2 cup black beans

-1/2 cup corn

-1/2 cup chopped tomatoes

-2 tablespoons olive oil

-1 teaspoon garlic, minced

-1/2 teaspoon ground cumin

-1/2 teaspoon chili powder

-Salt and pepper to taste

Instructions:

1. In a medium saucepan, bring 2 cups of water to a boil.

2. Add quinoa to the boiling water and reduce heat to low. Cook for 10-15 minutes, or until quinoa is cooked through.

3. In a separate pan, heat olive oil over medium heat.

4. Add garlic, cumin, and chili powder and cook for 1-2 minutes.

5. Add black beans, corn, and tomatoes and cook for an additional 5 minutes, stirring occasionally.

6. Season with salt and pepper, to taste.

7. Combine cooked quinoa and bean mixture in a bowl and serve.

Prep Time: 10 minutes

Cook Time: 20 minutes

Total Time: 30 minutes

Snack: Smoothie with banana, almond milk, and spinach

Ingredients:

- 1 banana
- 1 cup almond milk
- 1/2 cup spinach
- 2 tablespoons honey

Instructions:

1. Place the banana, almond milk, spinach and honey into a blender.

2. Blend until smooth.

3. Pour the smoothie into your desired glass and enjoy.

Prep Time: 5 minutes

Dinner: Grilled chicken with roasted vegetables and brown rice

Ingredients:
- 2 boneless and skinless chicken breasts
- 1 red bell pepper, chopped
- 1 green bell pepper, chopped
- 1 onion, chopped
- 2 cloves garlic, minced
- 2 tablespoons olive oil
- 2 teaspoons Italian seasoning

- 1 teaspoon salt
- 1/2 teaspoon pepper
- 1 cup brown rice
- 2 cups chicken broth

Instructions:

1. Preheat the oven to 400°F.

2. In a large bowl, combine the bell peppers, onion, garlic, olive oil, Italian seasoning, salt and pepper. Toss to combine.

3. Spread the vegetables on a baking sheet lined with parchment paper. Roast in a preheated oven for 20 minutes, stirring once halfway through.

4. Meanwhile, bring the chicken broth to a boil in a large saucepan over medium heat. Add the brown rice, reduce heat to low, cover and simmer for 20 minutes.

5. Heat a large skillet over medium-high heat. Add the chicken breasts and cook for 8-10 minutes, flipping once, until the chicken is cooked through.

6. To serve, divide the cooked brown rice among 4 plates. Top each with roasted vegetables and a chicken breast.

Prep Time: 10 minutes
Cook Time: 30 minutes

CHAPTER SIX

FERTILITY RECIPES

BREAKFAST

1. Apple Cinnamon Overnight Oats

Ingredients:

-1/2 cup rolled oats

-1/2 cup almond milk

-1/2 cup apples, diced

-1/2 teaspoon cinnamon

-1 teaspoon honey

Instructions:

In a bowl, combine the oats, almond milk, apples and cinnamon. Stir until combined.

Spoon the mixture into a container and cover with a lid. Place in the refrigerator overnight.

In the morning, sprinkle the oats with honey and enjoy.

Prep Time: 5 minutes

2. Avocado Toast

Ingredients:
- 1 slice of whole grain toast
- 1/4 avocado, sliced
- 1/4 teaspoon sea salt
- 1/4 teaspoon black pepper
- 1 teaspoon olive oil

Instructions:

Toast the slice of bread in a toaster or oven. Spread the avocado onto the toast and sprinkle with sea salt and pepper. Drizzle with olive oil.

Prep Time: 5 minutes

3. Banana Smoothie

Ingredients:
-1 banana
-1/2 cup almond milk
-1/4 teaspoon cinnamon
-1 teaspoon honey

Instructions:

Combine the banana, almond milk, cinnamon and honey in a blender. Blend until smooth.

Pour the smoothie into a glass and enjoy.

Prep Time: 5 minutes

4. Turmeric Tea

Ingredients:
-1 cup water
-1 teaspoon turmeric
-1 teaspoon honey
-Squeeze of lemon juice

Instructions:

Bring the water to a boil in a small pot. Add the turmeric and reduce the heat. Simmer for 5 minutes.

Strain the tea into a cup and stir in the honey and lemon juice. Enjoy.

Prep Time: 10 minutes

5. Egg Salad

Ingredients:
-4 eggs, boiled and chopped
-1/4 cup celery, diced
-1/4 cup onion, diced
-1/4 cup mayonnaise
-1/4 teaspoon sea salt
-1/4 teaspoon black pepper

Instructions:

In a bowl, combine the eggs, celery, onion, mayonnaise, salt and pepper. Mix until combined.

Serve the egg salad on toast or crackers.

Prep Time: 10 minutes

6. Berry Chia Pudding

Ingredients:

-1/4 cup chia seeds

-1 cup almond milk

-1 teaspoon honey

-1/2 cup mixed berries

Instructions:

In a bowl, combine the chia seeds, almond milk and honey. Stir until combined.

Cover the bowl with a lid and place in the refrigerator for at least 2 hours.

When ready to serve, top with the mixed berries and enjoy.

Prep Time: 5 minutes + 2 hours refrigeration time

7. Quinoa Salad

Ingredients:
-1 cup quinoa, cooked
-1/4 cup cherry tomatoes, diced
-1/4 cup cucumber, diced
-1/4 cup red onion, diced
-1/4 cup feta cheese
-1/4 cup olive oil
-1 tablespoon apple cider vinegar

-1 teaspoon oregano

Instructions:

In a bowl, combine the quinoa, tomatoes, cucumber, onion and feta cheese.

In a separate bowl, whisk together the olive oil, apple cider vinegar and oregano.

Pour the dressing over the quinoa mixture and stir until combined.

Prep Time: 10 minutes

8. Sweet Potato Toast

Ingredients:
-2 sweet potatoes, thinly sliced
-1 tablespoon olive oil
-1/4 teaspoon sea salt

-1/4 teaspoon black pepper

Instructions:

Preheat the oven to 400°F. Line a baking sheet with parchment paper.

Arrange the sweet potato slices on the baking sheet and brush with olive oil. Sprinkle it with sea salt and pepper.

Bake for 15 minutes, flipping halfway through.

Enjoy the sweet potato toast as is, or top with your favorite toppings.

Prep Time: 10 minutes

9. Zucchini Noodles

Ingredients:

-2 zucchinis, spiralized

-1 tablespoon olive oil

-1/4 teaspoon sea salt

-1/4 teaspoon black pepper

Instructions:

In a large skillet, heat the olive oil over medium-high heat.

Add the zucchini noodles and season with salt and pepper.

Cook for 5-7 minutes, stirring occasionally, until the noodles are tender.

Serve the zucchini noodles as is, or top with your favorite sauce.

Prep Time: 10 minutes

10. Green Smoothie

Ingredients:
-1/2 banana
-1/2 cup spinach
-1/2 cup almond milk
-1/2 teaspoon honey
-1/4 teaspoon cinnamon

Instructions:
Combine the banana, spinach, almond milk, honey and cinnamon in a blender. Blend until smooth.
Pour the smoothie into a glass and enjoy.

Prep Time: 5 minutes

11. Omelette

Ingredients:

-2 eggs

-1/4 cup red bell pepper, diced

-1/4 cup onion, diced

-1/4 teaspoon sea salt

-1/4 teaspoon black pepper

-1 teaspoon olive oil

Instructions:

In a bowl, whisk together the eggs, bell pepper, onion, salt and pepper.

Heat the olive oil in a large skillet over medium heat. Pour the egg mixture into the skillet and cook for 3-4 minutes. Flip the omelette and cook for an additional 3-4 minutes.

Slide the omelette onto a plate and enjoy.

Prep Time: 10 minutes

12. Hummus Toast

Ingredients:
-1 slice of whole grain toast
-2 tablespoons hummus
-1/4 cup cucumber, diced
-1/4 cup tomatoes, diced
-1/4 teaspoon oregano

Instructions:

Toast the slice of bread in a toaster or oven. Spread the hummus onto the toast and top with the cucumber, tomatoes and oregano. Enjoy the hummus toast.

Prep Time: 5 minutes

13. Greek Yogurt Parfait

Ingredients:

-1/2 cup plain Greek yogurt

-1/4 cup blueberries

-1/4 cup raspberries

-1 teaspoon honey

-1/4 teaspoon cinnamon

Instructions:

In a bowl, combine the yogurt, blueberries, raspberries, honey and cinnamon. Stir until combined.

Spoon the mixture into a jar or cup and enjoy.

Prep Time: 5 minutes

14. Chickpea Salad

Ingredients:
-1 can chickpeas, drained and rinsed
-1/4 cup celery, diced
-1/4 cup onion, diced
-1/4 cup mayonnaise
-1/4 teaspoon sea salt
-1/4 teaspoon black pepper

Instructions:

In a bowl, combine the chickpeas, celery, onion, mayonnaise, salt and pepper. Mix until combined.

Serve the chickpea salad on toast or crackers.

Prep Time: 10 minutes

15. Lentil Soup

Ingredients:

-1 tablespoon olive oil

-1/4 cup onion, diced

-1/4 cup celery, diced

-1/4 cup carrots, diced

-1 cup lentils

-4 cups vegetable broth

-1 teaspoon oregano

Instructions:

Heat the olive oil in a large pot over medium heat. Add the onion, celery and carrots and cook for 5 minutes.

Add the lentils and vegetable broth and bring to a boil. Reduce the heat, cover the pot and simmer for 20 minutes.

Stir in the oregano, season with salt and pepper and serve.

Prep Time: 25 minutes

LUNCH

1. Eggplant and Chickpea Curry

Ingredients:

- 2 tablespoons olive oil
- 2 cloves garlic, minced
- 1 onion, diced
- 1 teaspoon ground turmeric
- 1 teaspoon ground coriander
- 1 teaspoon ground cumin
- 1 teaspoon ground ginger
- 1/2 teaspoon ground cayenne pepper
- 1 large eggplant, diced
- 2 cups cooked chickpeas
- 1 (14-ounce) can diced tomatoes
- 1/2 cup vegetable broth
- 1/4 cup chopped fresh cilantro

Instructions:

1. Heat the oil in a large skillet over medium heat. Add the garlic and onion and cook until softened, about 5 minutes.

2. Stir in the turmeric, coriander, cumin, ginger, and cayenne pepper. Cook for 1 minute, stirring constantly.

3. Add the eggplant and cook until softened, about 5 minutes.

4. Stir in the chickpeas, tomatoes, and vegetable broth. Bring to a simmer, reduce the heat to low, and cook for 20 minutes.

5. Stir in the cilantro and season with salt and pepper to taste. Serve hot.

Prep Time: 15 minutes
Cook Time: 25 minutes

2. Burrito Bowl

Ingredients:
- 2 tablespoons olive oil
- 1 onion, diced
- 1 bell pepper, diced
- 1 teaspoon ground cumin
- 1 teaspoon chili powder
- 1/2 teaspoon garlic powder
- 1/2 teaspoon paprika
- 1/2 teaspoon ground coriander
- 1/2 teaspoon salt
- 1/4 teaspoon black pepper
- 1 (15-ounce) can black beans, drained and rinsed

- 2 cups cooked brown rice
- 2 cups shredded lettuce
- 1 cup salsa
- 1/2 cup shredded cheese
- 1/4 cup chopped fresh cilantro

Instructions:

1. Heat the oil in a large skillet over medium heat. Add the onion and bell pepper and cook until softened, about 5 minutes.

2. Stir in the cumin, chili powder, garlic powder, paprika, coriander, salt, and black pepper. Cook for 1 minute, stirring constantly.

3. Add the black beans and cook until heated through, about 5 minutes.

4. To assemble the burrito bowls, divide the rice among 4 bowls. Top each bowl with the lettuce, salsa, cheese, cilantro, and the black bean mixture.

Prep Time: 10 minutes
Cook Time: 10 minutes

3. Lentil Veggie Soup

Ingredients:
- 2 tablespoons olive oil
- 1 onion, diced
- 2 cloves garlic, minced
- 2 carrots, diced
- 2 celery stalks, diced
- 1 teaspoon ground cumin
- 1 teaspoon dried oregano

- 1 teaspoon dried thyme

- 1 teaspoon salt

- 1/4 teaspoon black pepper

- 1 (15-ounce) can diced tomatoes

- 4 cups vegetable broth

- 1 cup dried green lentils, rinsed and picked over

- 1/2 cup chopped fresh parsley

Instructions:

1. Heat the oil in a large pot over medium heat. Add the onion and garlic and cook until softened, about 5 minutes.

2. Stir in the carrots, celery, cumin, oregano, thyme, salt, and black pepper. Cook for 1 minute, stirring constantly.

3. Add the tomatoes, vegetable broth, and lentils and bring to a boil. Reduce the heat to low and simmer for 20 minutes, or until the lentils are tender.

4. Stir in the parsley and season with salt and pepper to taste. Serve hot.

Prep Time: 10 minutes
Cook Time: 30 minutes

4. Baked Tofu

Ingredients:
- 1 (16-ounce) package extra-firm tofu, drained and pressed
- 2 tablespoons olive oil
- 2 tablespoons tamari

- 1 tablespoon maple syrup

- 1 tablespoon apple cider vinegar

- 1 tablespoon sesame oil

- 1 teaspoon garlic powder

- 1/2 teaspoon ground ginger

Instructions:

1. Preheat the oven to 375°F.
2. Cut the tofu into cubes and place in a large bowl.
3. In a small bowl, whisk together the olive oil, tamari, maple syrup, apple cider vinegar, sesame oil, garlic powder, and ginger.
4. Pour the marinade over the tofu and gently toss to coat.
5. Spread the tofu in a single layer on a baking sheet lined with parchment paper.

6. Bake for 25 minutes, or until golden brown and crispy.

Prep Time: 10 minutes
Cook Time: 25 minutes

5. Quinoa Salad

Ingredients:
- 2 cups cooked quinoa
- 1/2 cup diced red onion
- 1/2 cup diced red bell pepper
- 1/2 cup diced cucumber
- 1/2 cup crumbled feta cheese
- 1/4 cup chopped fresh parsley
- 2 tablespoons olive oil
- 2 tablespoons lemon juice
- 1 teaspoon dried oregano

- Salt and pepper to taste

Instructions:

1. In a large bowl, combine the quinoa, red onion, bell pepper, cucumber, feta cheese, and parsley.

2. In a small bowl, whisk together the olive oil, lemon juice, oregano, salt, and pepper.

3. Pour the dressing over the quinoa mixture and toss to combine.

4. Serve chilled or at room temperature.

Prep Time: 10 minutes

Cook Time: 0 minutes

6. Veggie Sandwich

Ingredients:

- 4 slices whole wheat bread

- 2 tablespoons hummus
- 1/4 cup shredded carrots
- 1/4 cup sliced cucumber
- 1/4 cup alfalfa sprouts
- 1/4 cup shredded cheese

Instructions:

1. Spread the hummus on the bread slices.

2. Top 2 of the slices with the carrots, cucumber, sprouts, and cheese.

3. Top with the remaining bread slices.

4. Cut the sandwiches in half and serve.

Prep Time: 5 minutes
Cook Time: 0 minutes

7. Chickpea Salad

Ingredients:

- 2 (15-ounce) cans chickpeas, drained and rinsed
- 1/2 cup diced red onion
- 1/2 cup diced red bell pepper
- 1/2 cup diced cucumber
- 1/4 cup crumbled feta cheese
- 2 tablespoons olive oil
- 2 tablespoons lemon juice
- 1 teaspoon dried oregano
- Salt and pepper to taste

Instructions:

1. In a large bowl, combine the chickpeas, red onion, bell pepper, cucumber, and feta cheese.

2. In a small bowl, whisk together the olive oil, lemon juice, oregano, salt, and pepper.

3. Pour the dressing over the chickpea mixture and toss to combine.

4. Serve chilled or at room temperature.

Prep Time: 10 minutes
Cook Time: 0 minutes

8. Mediterranean Pasta Salad

Ingredients:

- 8 ounces whole wheat pasta
- 1/2 cup diced red onion
- 1/2 cup diced red bell pepper
- 1/2 cup diced cucumber
- 1/2 cup crumbled feta cheese
- 1/4 cup kalamata olives, pitted and halved
- 2 tablespoons olive oil
- 2 tablespoons lemon juice
- 1 teaspoon dried oregano
- Salt and pepper to taste

Instructions:

1. Cook the pasta according to package instructions. Drain and set aside.

2. In a large bowl, combine the pasta, red onion, bell pepper, cucumber, feta cheese and olives.

3. In a small bowl, whisk together the olive oil, lemon juice, oregano, salt, and pepper.

4. Pour the dressing over the pasta mixture and toss to combine.

5. Serve chilled or at room temperature.

Prep Time: 10 minutes
Cook Time: 10 minutes

9. Falafel

Ingredients:

- 1 (15-ounce) can chickpeas, drained and rinsed
- 1/2 onion, diced
- 3 cloves garlic, minced
- 1/2 cup fresh parsley, chopped
- 1/4 cup fresh cilantro, chopped
- 1 teaspoon ground cumin
- 1 teaspoon ground coriander
- 1/2 teaspoon baking powder
- 1/2 teaspoon salt
- 1/4 teaspoon black pepper
- 2 tablespoons olive oil
- 2 tablespoons all-purpose flour

Instructions:

1. Preheat the oven to 375°F. Line a baking sheet with parchment paper.

2. In a food processor, combine the chickpeas, onion, garlic, parsley, cilantro, cumin, coriander, baking powder, salt, and pepper. Pulse until combined but still chunky.

3. Transfer the mixture to a bowl and stir in the olive oil and flour.

4. Form the mixture into small patties and place on the prepared baking sheet.

5. Bake for 20 minutes, flipping halfway through.

Prep Time: 10 minutes
Cook Time: 20 minutes

10. Chinese Fried Rice

Ingredients:
- 2 tablespoons vegetable oil
- 1 onion, diced
- 2 cloves garlic, minced
- 2 carrots, diced
- 1 cup frozen peas
- 2 cups cooked brown rice
- 2 tablespoons tamari
- 2 tablespoons rice vinegar
- 1 teaspoon sesame oil

Instructions:

1. Heat the vegetable oil in a large skillet over medium heat. Add the onion and garlic and cook until softened, about 5 minutes.

2. Add the carrots and peas and cook for 5 minutes.

3. Add the cooked rice and stir to combine.

4. Stir in the tamari, rice vinegar, and sesame oil. Cook until heated through, about 5 minutes.

5. Serve hot.

Prep Time: 10 minutes
Cook Time: 15 minutes

11. Curried Vegetable Bowl

Ingredients:
- 2 tablespoons olive oil

- 1 onion, diced
- 1 bell pepper, diced
- 2 cloves garlic, minced
- 1 teaspoon ground cumin
- 1 teaspoon curry powder
- 1 teaspoon ground ginger
- 1/2 teaspoon ground coriander
- 1/2 teaspoon salt
- 1/4 teaspoon black pepper
- 1 (15-ounce) can chickpeas, drained and rinsed
- 2 cups cooked brown rice
- 1/4 cup chopped fresh cilantro

Instructions:

1. Heat the oil in a large skillet over medium heat. Add the onion and bell pepper and cook until softened, about 5 minutes.

2. Stir in the garlic, cumin, curry powder, ginger, coriander, salt, and black pepper. Cook for 1 minute, stirring constantly.

3. Add the chickpeas and cook until heated through, about 5 minutes.

4. To assemble the bowls, divide the rice among 4 bowls. Top each bowl with the chickpea mixture and cilantro.

Prep Time: 10 minutes
Cook Time: 10 minutes

12. Avocado Toast

Ingredients:
- 4 slices whole wheat bread

- 2 avocados, mashed
- 2 tablespoons olive oil
- 2 tablespoons lemon juice
- 1/4 teaspoon garlic powder
- Salt and pepper to taste

Instructions:

1. Toast the bread slices.

2. In a small bowl, whisk together the avocado, olive oil, lemon juice, garlic powder, salt, and pepper.

3. Spread the mashed avocado on the toasted bread slices.

4. Sprinkle it with salt and pepper to taste.

Prep Time: 5 minutes

Cook Time: 5 minutes

13. Lentil Tacos

Ingredients:
- 2 tablespoons olive oil
- 1 onion, diced
- 1 bell pepper, diced
- 2 cloves garlic, minced
- 1 teaspoon ground cumin
- 1 teaspoon chili powder
- 1 teaspoon dried oregano
- 1/2 teaspoon ground coriander
- 1/2 teaspoon salt
- 1/4 teaspoon black pepper
- 1 (15-ounce) can lentils, drained and rinsed
- 8 tacos shells

- 1/2 cup salsa

Instructions:

1. Heat the oil in a large skillet over medium heat. Add the onion and bell pepper and cook until softened, about 5 minutes.

2. Stir in the garlic, cumin, chili powder, oregano, coriander, salt, and black pepper. Cook for 1 minute, stirring constantly.

3. Add the lentils and cook until heated through, about 5 minutes.

4. To assemble the tacos, divide the lentil mixture among the taco shells. Top with the salsa.

Prep Time: 10 minutes

Cook Time: 10 minutes

14. Stir-Fried Veggies

Ingredients:

- 2 tablespoons vegetable oil
- 1 onion, diced
- 2 cloves garlic, minced
- 2 carrots, sliced
- 1 bell pepper, sliced
- 1 cup snow peas
- 1 cup mushrooms, sliced
- 2 tablespoons tamari
- 2 tablespoons rice vinegar
- 1 teaspoon sesame oil

Instructions:

1. Heat the oil in a large skillet over medium heat. Add the onion and garlic and cook until softened, about 5 minutes.

2. Add the carrots, bell pepper, snow peas, and mushrooms and cook until tender, about 5 minutes.

3. Stir in the tamari, rice vinegar, and sesame oil. Cook until heated through, about 5 minutes.

4. Serve hot.

Prep Time: 10 minutes
Cook Time: 10 minutes

15. Tempeh Stir-Fry

Ingredients:

- 2 tablespoons vegetable oil
- 1 onion, diced
- 2 cloves garlic, minced
- 1 (8-ounce) package tempeh, cut into cubes
- 2 carrots, sliced
- 1 bell pepper, sliced
- 1 cup snow peas
- 1 cup mushrooms, sliced
- 2 tablespoons tamari
- 2 tablespoons rice vinegar

Instructions:

1. Heat the oil in a large skillet over medium heat. Add the onion and garlic and cook until softened, about 5 minutes.

2. Add the tempeh and cook and cook until lightly browned, about 5 minutes.

3. Add the carrots, bell pepper, snow peas, and mushrooms and cook until tender, about 5 minutes.

4. Stir in the tamari and rice vinegar. Cook until heated through, about 5 minutes.

5. Serve hot.

Prep Time: 10 minutes
Cook Time: 15 minutes

DINNER

1. Quinoa Stuffed Peppers (30 minutes):

Ingredients:
- 4 bell peppers
- 2 tablespoons olive oil
- 1 onion, diced
- 2 cloves garlic, minced
- 2 carrots, diced
- 1 cup cooked quinoa
- 1/2 cup corn
- 1/2 cup cooked black beans
- 1/4 teaspoon chili powder
- 1/4 teaspoon cumin
- 1/4 teaspoon salt
- 1/4 teaspoon pepper
- 1/2 cup shredded cheddar cheese

Instructions:

1. Preheat the oven to 350°F.

2. Cut the tops off the bell peppers and remove the insides. Place in a baking dish.

3. In a large skillet, heat olive oil over medium heat.

4. Add onion, garlic, and carrots and sauté for about 5 minutes or until onions are translucent.

5. Add cooked quinoa, corn, black beans, chili powder, cumin, salt, and pepper. Stir to combine.

6. Spoon the quinoa mixture into the bell peppers. Top with shredded cheese.

7. Bake for 30 minutes or until peppers are tender.

2. Zucchini Noodle Stir Fry (20 minutes):

Ingredients:
- 2 tablespoons sesame oil
- 1 onion, diced
- 1 red bell pepper, diced
- 2 cloves garlic, minced
- 2 carrots, diced
- 1 zucchini, spiralized
- 1 cup cooked edamame
- 2 tablespoons soy sauce
- 1/4 teaspoon ground ginger

Instructions:

1. Heat sesame oil in a large skillet over medium-high heat.

2. Add onion, bell pepper, garlic, and carrots and sauté for about 5 minutes.

3. Add zucchini noodles and edamame and sauté for another 5 minutes.

4. Add soy sauce and ground ginger and stir to combine.

5. Cook for an additional 5 minutes until vegetables are tender.

3. Lentil and Sweet Potato Curry (35 minutes):

Ingredients:

- 1 tablespoon olive oil
- 1 onion, diced
- 2 cloves garlic, minced
- 1 tablespoon minced ginger
- 1 tablespoon curry powder
- 1/2 teaspoon ground cumin
- 1/4 teaspoon turmeric
- 1 sweet potato, cubed
- 1 cup cooked lentils
- 1 can (14.5 ounces) coconut milk
- 1/4 teaspoon salt

Instructions:

1. Heat olive oil in a large skillet over medium heat.

2. Add onion, garlic, and ginger and sauté for about 5 minutes.

3. Add curry powder, cumin, and turmeric and sauté for another 2 minutes.

4. Add sweet potato, lentils, coconut milk, and salt and stir to combine.

5. Simmer for about 20 minutes or until sweet potatoes are tender.

4. Baked Salmon with Creamy Dill Sauce (25 minutes):

Ingredients:
- 2 tablespoons olive oil
- 4 salmon fillets

- 1/2 teaspoon salt

- 1/4 teaspoon pepper

- 1/2 cup plain Greek yogurt

- 2 tablespoons minced dill

- 1 tablespoon lemon juice

Instructions:

1. Preheat the oven to 400°F.

2. Grease a baking dish with olive oil and place salmon fillets in the dish. Sprinkle it with salt and pepper.

3. Bake for 20 minutes or until salmon is cooked through.

4. Meanwhile, in a small bowl, mix together Greek yogurt, dill, and lemon juice.

5. Serve salmon with creamy dill sauce.

5. Eggplant Parmesan (45 minutes):

Ingredients:
- 2 tablespoons olive oil
- 1 eggplant, sliced into 1/4-inch slices
- 1/2 teaspoon salt
- 1/4 teaspoon pepper
- 1 cup marinara sauce
- 1 cup shredded mozzarella cheese
- 1/4 cup grated Parmesan cheese
- Fresh basil, for garnish

Instructions:
1. Preheat the oven to 375°F.

2. Grease a baking sheet with olive oil and place eggplant slices on the sheet. Sprinkle it with salt and pepper.

3. Bake for 20 minutes or until the eggplant is tender.

4. Spread marinara sauce over the eggplant slices and top with mozzarella and Parmesan cheese.

5. Bake for an additional 20 minutes or until the cheese is melted and bubbly.

6. Garnish with fresh basil.

6. Roasted Vegetable Bowl (30 minutes):

Ingredients:

- 2 tablespoons olive oil
- 1 head cauliflower, cut into florets
- 1 red bell pepper, sliced
- 1 onion, sliced
- 2 cloves garlic, minced
- 1/2 teaspoon salt
- 1/4 teaspoon pepper
- 1 cup cooked quinoa
- 1/4 cup chopped parsley

Instructions:

1. Preheat the oven to 400°F.

2. Grease a baking sheet with olive oil and add cauliflower, bell pepper, onion, and garlic. Sprinkle it with salt and pepper.

3. Roast for 20 minutes or until vegetables are tender.

4. Place roasted vegetables in a bowl with cooked quinoa and chopped parsley.

5. Serve warm.

7. Roasted Chickpea and Carrot Salad (30 minutes):

Ingredients:
- 2 tablespoons olive oil
- 1 can (15 ounces) chickpeas, drained and rinsed
- 2 carrots, peeled and sliced
- 1/2 teaspoon salt
- 1/4 teaspoon pepper

- 1/4 cup chopped parsley
- 2 tablespoons lemon juice

Instructions:

1. Preheat the oven to 400°F.

2. Grease a baking sheet with olive oil and add chickpeas and carrots. Sprinkle it with salt and pepper.

3. Roast for 20 minutes or until vegetables are tender.

4. Place roasted vegetables in a bowl with chopped parsley and lemon juice.

5. Serve warm.

8. Avocado Toast (10 minutes):

Ingredients:
- 2 slices whole grain bread
- 2 tablespoons olive oil
- 1 avocado, mashed
- 1/4 teaspoon salt
- 1/4 teaspoon pepper

Instructions:
1. Toast the bread in a toaster.

2. Brush the toast with olive oil.

3. Top with mashed avocado and sprinkle with salt and pepper.

4. Serve warm.

9. Broccoli and Cauliflower Soup (30 minutes):

Ingredients:
- 2 tablespoons olive oil
- 1 onion, diced
- 2 cloves garlic, minced
- 1 head broccoli, cut into florets
- 1 head cauliflower, cut into florets
- 4 cups vegetable broth
- 1/2 teaspoon salt
- 1/4 teaspoon pepper

Instructions:
1. Heat olive oil in a large pot over medium heat.

2. Add onion and garlic and sauté for about 5 minutes.

3. Add broccoli, cauliflower, and vegetable broth and bring to a simmer.

4. Simmer for 20 minutes or until vegetables are tender.

5. Puree the soup in a blender or food processor until smooth.

6. Serve warm.

10. Stuffed Acorn Squash (45 minutes):

Ingredients:
- 2 tablespoons olive oil

- 2 acorn squash, halved and seeded
- 1 onion, diced
- 2 cloves garlic, minced
- 2 carrots, diced
- 1 cup cooked quinoa
- 1/2 cup corn
- 1/2 cup cooked black beans
- 1/4 teaspoon chili powder
- 1/4 teaspoon cumin
- 1/4 teaspoon salt
- 1/4 teaspoon pepper
- 1/2 cup shredded cheddar cheese

Instructions:

1. Preheat the oven to 375°F.

2. Grease a baking dish with olive oil and add acorn squash halves.

3. In a large skillet, heat olive oil over medium heat.

4. Add onion, garlic, and carrots and sauté for about 5 minutes or until onions are translucent.

5. Add cooked quinoa, corn, black beans, chili powder, cumin, salt, and pepper. Stir to combine.

6. Spoon the quinoa mixture into the squash halves. Top with shredded cheese.

7. Bake for 30 minutes or until squash is tender.

11. Lentil and Kale Salad (20 minutes):

Ingredients:

- 2 tablespoons olive oil
- 1 onion, diced
- 2 cloves garlic, minced
- 1 cup cooked lentils
- 2 cups chopped kale
- 1/4 teaspoon salt
- 1/4 teaspoon pepper
- 2 tablespoons lemon juice

Instructions:

1. Heat olive oil in a large skillet over medium heat.

2. Add onion and garlic and sauté for about 5 minutes.

3. Add lentils, kale, salt, and pepper and sauté for an additional 5 minutes.

4. Remove from heat and stir in lemon juice.

5. Serve warm or cold.

12. Zucchini Lasagna (45 minutes):

Ingredients:
- 2 tablespoons olive oil
- 1 onion, diced
- 2 cloves garlic, minced
- 1 zucchini, sliced
- 1 red bell pepper, diced
- 1 eggplant, diced
- 1 can (14.5 ounces) diced tomatoes
- 1/2 teaspoon salt

- 1/4 teaspoon pepper

- 1/4 teaspoon oregano

- 1/4 teaspoon basil

- 1 cup ricotta cheese

- 1 cup shredded mozzarella cheese

Instructions:

1. Preheat the oven to 375°F.

2. Grease a 9x13 inch baking dish with olive oil.

3. In a large skillet, heat olive oil over medium heat.

4. Add onion, garlic, zucchini, and bell pepper and sauté for about 5 minutes.

5. Add diced tomatoes, salt, pepper, oregano, and basil and stir to combine.

6. Spread the tomato mixture in the prepared baking dish.

7. Top with ricotta cheese and mozzarella cheese.

8. Bake for 30 minutes or until the cheese is melted and bubbly.

13. Baked Falafel (30 minutes):

Ingredients:
- 2 tablespoons olive oil
- 2 cans (15 ounces) chickpeas, drained and rinsed

- 1 onion, diced
- 2 cloves garlic, minced
- 1/2 teaspoon salt
- 1/4 teaspoon pepper
- 1 teaspoon ground cumin
- 2 tablespoons chopped parsley

Instructions:

1. Preheat the oven to 375°F.

2. Grease a baking sheet with olive oil.

3. Place chickpeas, onion, garlic, salt, pepper, cumin, and parsley in a food processor and pulse until mixture is combined but still slightly chunky.

4. Form mixture into small patties and place on a prepared baking sheet.

5. Bake for 20 minutes or until firm and golden brown.

14. Sweet Potato Black Bean Burrito Bowl (30 minutes):

Ingredients:
- 2 tablespoons olive oil
- 1 onion, diced
- 2 cloves garlic, minced
- 1 sweet potato, cubed
- 1 can (15 ounces) black beans, drained and rinsed
- 1 teaspoon chili powder
- 1/2 teaspoon cumin

- 1/4 teaspoon salt
- 1/4 teaspoon pepper
- 2 cups cooked quinoa
- 1/4 cup chopped cilantro

Instructions:

1. Heat olive oil in a large skillet over medium heat.

2. Add onion, garlic, and sweet potato and sauté for about 5 minutes.

3. Add black beans, chili powder, cumin, salt, and pepper and stir to combine.

4. Simmer for about 10 minutes or until the sweet potato is tender.

5. Serve mixture over cooked quinoa and top with chopped cilantro.

15. Asparagus Quiche (45 minutes):

Ingredients:
- 2 tablespoons olive oil
- 1 onion, diced
- 2 cloves garlic, minced
- 1 bunch asparagus, cut into 1-inch pieces
- 1/2 teaspoon salt
- 1/4 teaspoon pepper
- 1 cup shredded mozzarella cheese
- 4 eggs
- 1/2 cup milk

Instructions:
1. Preheat the oven to 375°F.

2. Grease a 9-inch pie plate with olive oil.

3. In a large skillet, heat olive oil over medium heat.

4. Add onion, garlic, and asparagus and sauté for about 5 minutes.

5. Spread the asparagus mixture in the prepared pie plate. Sprinkle it with salt, pepper, and mozzarella cheese.

6. In a medium bowl, whisk together eggs and milk.

7. Pour egg mixture over the asparagus mixture.

8. Bake for 30 minutes or until eggs are set.

SNACK

1. Avocado and Egg Fertility Snack:

Introduction: This creamy, protein-packed snack is a great way to boost your fertility. Avocados are high in folate and healthy fats, while eggs are a great source of choline, which has been linked to increased fertility.

Ingredients:
-1 ripe avocado
-2 hard-boiled eggs
-Salt and pepper to taste

Instructions:

1. Peel and mash the avocado into a bowl.

2. Peel and chop the hard-boiled eggs, then add them to the mashed avocado.

3. Mix together and season with salt and pepper to taste.

4. Serve as a dip or spread on toast or crackers.

Prep Time: 10 minutes

2. Fertility Trail Mix:

Introduction: This easy-to-make trail mix is full of fertility-boosting ingredients like pumpkin seeds, sunflower seeds, dried fruit, and nuts.

Ingredients:
- ½ cup pumpkin seeds
- ½ cup sunflower seeds
- ½ cup dried cranberries
- ½ cup dried apricots
- ½ cup almonds
- ½ cup walnuts
- ¼ cup dark chocolate chips

Instructions:
1. Combine all the ingredients in a bowl and mix together.

2. Divide into individual portions and store in airtight containers.

3. Enjoy as a snack or add to yogurt or oatmeal.

Prep Time: 10 minutes

3. Fertility Smoothie Bowl:

Introduction: This smoothie bowl is a great way to get some of the key nutrients needed for fertility.
The combination of banana, mango, and almond milk provide a good balance of protein, healthy fats, and carbohydrates.

Ingredients:

-1 banana
-1 cup frozen mango

-1 cup almond milk

-1 tbsp chia seeds

-1 tbsp hemp seeds

-1 tbsp almond butter

-1 tsp honey

Instructions:

1. Place all ingredients in a blender and blend until smooth.

2. Pour mixture into a bowl and top with desired toppings.

3. Enjoy immediately or store in an airtight container for later.

Prep Time: 10 minutes

4. Fertility Power Bowl:

Introduction: This nutrient-packed power bowl is full of fertility-boosting ingredients like quinoa, sweet potatoes, spinach, and eggs.

Ingredients:
-1 cup cooked quinoa
-1 cup roasted sweet potatoes
-½ cup cooked spinach
-2 hard-boiled eggs
-Salt and pepper to taste

Instructions:

1. Place the quinoa in a bowl and top with the roasted sweet potatoes and cooked spinach.

2. Peel and chop the hard-boiled eggs, then add to the bowl.

3. Season with salt and pepper to taste and serve.

Prep Time: 15 minutes

5. Fertility Granola Bars:

Introduction: These easy-to-make granola bars are packed with fertility-boosting ingredients like oats, nuts, and dried fruit.

Ingredients:

-2 cups rolled oats
-1 cup nuts (almonds, walnuts, or pecans)
-½ cup dried cranberries or raisins
-½ cup honey
-2 tbsp melted coconut oil
-1 tsp vanilla extract

Instructions:

1. Preheat the oven to 350 degrees F.

2. In a bowl, mix together the oats, nuts, and dried fruit.

3. In a separate bowl, mix together the honey, coconut oil, and vanilla extract.

4. Combine the wet and dry ingredients and mix until thoroughly combined.

5. Spread the mixture onto a baking sheet lined with parchment paper and press into an even layer.

6. Bake for 20-25 minutes until golden brown.

7. Let cool before cutting into bars.

Prep Time: 25 minutes

6. Fertility Hummus:

Introduction: This creamy hummus is a great way to get some of the nutrients needed for fertility. The combination of chickpeas, tahini, and olive oil provide a good balance of protein, fiber, and healthy fats.

Ingredients:

-2 cups cooked chickpeas
-¼ cup tahini
-¼ cup olive oil
-2 cloves garlic
-Juice of 1 lemon
-Salt and pepper to taste

Instructions:
1. Place all ingredients in a food processor and blend until smooth.

2. Taste and adjust seasoning as needed.

3. Serve with crackers or vegetables.

Prep Time: 10 minutes

7. Fertility Energy Balls:

Introduction: These no-bake energy balls are a great way to get some of the key nutrients needed for fertility.
The combination of nuts, seeds, and dried fruit provide a good balance of protein, healthy fats, and carbohydrates.

Ingredients:
-1 cup almonds
-1 cup walnuts

-½ cup pumpkin seeds

-½ cup sunflower seeds

-½ cup dried cranberries or raisins

-½ cup dates, pitted and chopped

-2 tbsp chia seeds

-2 tbsp hemp seeds

-1/3 cup almond butter

-2 tbsp honey

Instructions:

1. Place all the ingredients in a food processor and blend until mixture is combined and forms a dough.

2. Roll into balls and store in an airtight container in the refrigerator.

3. Enjoy as a snack or add to yogurt or oatmeal.

Prep Time: 15 minutes

8. Fertility Popcorn:

Introduction: This popcorn is a delicious and easy way to get some of the key nutrients needed for fertility.

The combination of nuts, seeds, and dried fruit provide a good balance of protein, healthy fats, and carbohydrates.

Ingredients:
- ¼ cup popcorn kernels
- 2 tbsp coconut oil
- ¼ cup almonds
- ¼ cup walnuts
- ¼ cup pumpkin seeds

-¼ cup sunflower seeds

-¼ cup dried cranberries or raisins

-¼ cup honey

-Salt to taste

Instructions:

1. Heat the coconut oil in a large pot over medium heat.

2. Add the popcorn kernels and cover the pot with a lid.

3. Cook for 3-4 minutes or until popcorn has popped.

4. Transfer the popcorn to a large bowl and add the nuts, seeds, and dried fruit.

5. Drizzle with honey and season with salt to taste.

6. Mix together and enjoy.

Prep Time: 10 minutes

9. Fertility Smoothie:

Introduction: This smoothie is a great way to get some of the key nutrients needed for fertility.
The combination of banana, spinach, and almond milk provide a good balance of protein, healthy fats, and carbohydrates.

Ingredients:
-1 banana

-1 cup almond milk

-1 cup spinach

-1 tbsp chia seeds

-1 tbsp hemp seeds

-1 tbsp almond butter

-1 tsp honey

Instructions:

1. Place all ingredients in a blender and blend until smooth.

2. Pour into a glass and enjoy immediately.

Prep Time: 5 minutes

10. Fertility Yogurt Parfait:

Introduction: This yogurt parfait is a great way to get some of the key nutrients needed for fertility.

The combination of Greek yogurt, nuts, and fruit provide a good balance of protein, healthy fats, and carbohydrates.

Ingredients:

-2 cups plain Greek yogurt

-½ cup almonds

-½ cup walnuts

-½ cup dried cranberries or raisins

-½ cup blueberries

-½ cup sliced strawberries

Instructions:

1. Place the yogurt in a bowl and top with the almonds, walnuts, and dried fruit.

2. Top with the blueberries and strawberries.

3. Enjoy as a snack or breakfast.

Prep Time: 5 minutes

11. Fertility Kale Chips:

Introduction: These delicious kale chips are a great way to get some of the key nutrients needed for fertility.

The combination of kale, olive oil, and sea salt provide a good balance of vitamins, minerals, and antioxidants.

Ingredients:

-1 bunch kale, washed and dried

-2 tbsp olive oil

-1 tsp sea salt

Instructions:

1. Preheat the oven to 350 degrees F.

2. Place the kale on a baking sheet and drizzle with the olive oil.

3. Sprinkle with the sea salt and mix together until kale is evenly coated.

4. Bake for 10-15 minutes until kale is crispy.

5. Enjoy as a snack or side dish.

Prep Time: 10 minutes

12. Fertility Fruit Salad:

Introduction: This fruit salad is a great way to get some of the key nutrients needed for fertility.
The combination of apples, oranges, bananas, and dates provide a good balance of vitamins, minerals, and antioxidants.

Ingredients:
-2 apples, cored and diced
-2 oranges, peeled and diced
-2 bananas, sliced
-½ cup dates, pitted and chopped
-2 tbsp honey
-Juice of 1 lemon

Instructions:

1. Place the apples, oranges, bananas, and dates in a bowl and mix together.

2. In a separate bowl, mix together the honey and lemon juice.

3. Pour the honey mixture over the fruit and mix together.

4. Enjoy as a snack or dessert.

Prep Time: 10 minutes

13. Fertility Trail Mix Bars:

Introduction: These easy-to-make trail mix bars are full of fertility-boosting ingredients like oats, nuts, and dried fruit.

Ingredients:
- 2 cups rolled oats
- 1 cup almonds
- ½ cup pumpkin seeds
- ½ cup sunflower seeds
- ½ cup dried cranberries or raisins
- ½ cup honey
- 2 tbsp melted coconut oil
- 1 tsp vanilla extract

Instructions:
1. Preheat the oven to 350 degrees F.

2. In a bowl, mix together the oats, nuts, and dried fruit.

3. In a separate bowl, mix together the honey, coconut oil, and vanilla extract.

4. Combine the wet and dry ingredients and mix until thoroughly combined.

5. Spread the mixture onto a baking sheet lined with parchment paper and press into an even layer.

6. Bake for 20-25 minutes until golden brown.

7. Let cool before cutting into bars.

Prep Time: 25 minutes

14. Fertility Protein Balls:

Introduction: These no-bake protein balls are a great way to get some of the key nutrients needed for fertility.
The combination of nuts, seeds, and nut butter provide a good balance of protein, healthy fats, and carbohydrates.

Ingredients:
-1 cup almonds
-1 cup walnuts
-½ cup pumpkin seeds
-½ cup sunflower seeds
-½ cup almond butter
-2 tbsp honey
-1 tsp vanilla extract.

Instructions:

1. Place all the ingredients in a food processor and blend until mixture is combined and forms a dough.

2. Roll into balls and store in an airtight container in the refrigerator.

3. Enjoy as a snack or add to yogurt or oatmeal.

Prep Time: 15 minutes

15. Fertility Overnight Oats:

Introduction: This delicious overnight oats recipe is a great way to get some of the key nutrients needed for fertility.

The combination of oats, nuts, and dried fruit provide a good balance of protein, healthy fats, and carbohydrates.

Ingredients:
- 2 cups rolled oats
- 2 cups almond milk
- ½ cup almonds
- ½ cup walnuts
- ½ cup dried cranberries or raisins
- 2 tbsp chia seeds
- 2 tbsp hemp seeds
- 1 tsp honey

Instructions:

1. Place the oats and almond milk in a bowl and mix together.

2. Add the almonds, walnuts, and dried fruit and mix together.

3. Add the chia seeds, hemp seeds, and honey and mix together.

4. Cover and refrigerate overnight.

5. Enjoy as a snack or breakfast.

Prep Time: 10 minutes

DESSERT

1. Peach Cobbler

Ingredients:

3 cups of fresh peaches, peeled, sliced

1/4 cup of butter

1 cup of self-rising flour

1 cup of white sugar

1 cup of milk

Instructions:

1. Preheat your oven to 375 degrees Fahrenheit.

2. Place the peaches in a 9x13 inch baking dish.

3. In a medium bowl, mix together the butter, flour, sugar, and milk until well combined.

4. Pour the mixture over the peaches and spread evenly.

5. Bake in a preheated oven for approximately 30 minutes until the top is golden brown.

Prep Time: 15 minutes
Cook Time: 30 minutes
Total Time: 45 minutes

2. Lemon Meringue Pie

Ingredients:

1 9-inch pre-made graham cracker pie crust

3 eggs, separated

1/2 cup of white sugar

3 tablespoons of all-purpose flour

1/4 teaspoon of salt

1 cup of water

1/4 cup of lemon juice

3 tablespoons of butter

Instructions:

1. Preheat the oven to 375 degrees Fahrenheit.

2. In a medium bowl, beat the egg whites until soft peaks form.

3. In a separate bowl, combine the sugar, flour, and salt.

4. Gradually add the water, lemon juice, and butter to the sugar mixture.

5. Pour the mixture into the egg whites and beat until light and fluffy.

6. Pour into the graham cracker pie crust and bake for 25 minutes or until the top is golden brown.

Prep Time: 15 minutes
Cook Time: 25 minutes

Total Time: 40 minutes

3. Chocolate Cake

Ingredients:

2 cups of all-purpose flour

2 cups of white sugar

1 teaspoon of baking soda

1 teaspoon of salt

1 cup of cocoa powder

1 cup of boiling water

1 cup of buttermilk

2 eggs

1/2 cup of vegetable oil

1 teaspoon of vanilla extract

Instructions:

1. Preheat the oven to 350 degrees Fahrenheit.

2. Grease and flour a 9x13 inch baking pan.

3. In a large bowl, mix together the flour, sugar, baking soda, salt, and cocoa powder.

4. Add the boiling water, buttermilk, eggs, oil, and vanilla extract. Beat until smooth.

5. Pour batter into the prepared pan and bake for 30-35 minutes or until a toothpick inserted into the center comes out clean.

Prep Time: 15 minutes
Cook Time: 30-35 minutes
Total Time: 45-50 minutes

4. Apple Pie

Ingredients:

2 9-inch unbaked pie crusts

6 cups of thinly sliced apples

1/2 cup of white sugar

1/2 cup of brown sugar

3 tablespoons of all-purpose flour

1 teaspoon of ground cinnamon

1/4 teaspoon of ground nutmeg

6 tablespoons of butter

Instructions:

1. Preheat the oven to 425 degrees Fahrenheit.

2. Place one of the pie crusts in the bottom of a 9-inch pie plate.

3. In a large bowl, mix together the apples, sugars, flour, cinnamon, and nutmeg.

4. Pour the mixture into the pie crust and dot with butter.

5. Place the second crust on top of the pie and seal the edges. Cut a few slits in the top.

6. Bake in a preheated oven for 40-50 minutes or until golden brown.

Prep Time: 15 minutes
Cook Time: 40-50 minutes
Total Time: 55-65 minutes

5. Pecan Pie

Ingredients:

1 9-inch unbaked pie crust

3 eggs, beaten

1 cup of dark corn syrup

1 cup of white sugar

2 tablespoons of melted butter

1 teaspoon of vanilla extract

1 cup of chopped pecans

Instructions:

1. Preheat the oven to 350 degrees Fahrenheit.

2. Place the pie crust in a 9-inch pie plate.

3. In a medium bowl, mix together the eggs, corn syrup, sugar, butter, and vanilla extract.

4. Stir in the pecans and pour the mixture into the pie crust.

5. Bake in a preheated oven for 40-50 minutes or until golden brown.

Prep Time: 15 minutes
Cook Time: 40-50 minutes
Total Time: 55-65 minutes

6. Banana Pudding

Ingredients:
3 cups of cold milk

1 package of instant vanilla pudding mix

3 ripe bananas, sliced

1/2 teaspoon of ground cinnamon

1/2 teaspoon of ground nutmeg

1 9-inch pre-made graham cracker crust

Instructions:

1. In a medium bowl, combine the milk and pudding mix. Beat until thick.

2. Add the bananas, cinnamon, and nutmeg. Stir until well combined.

3. Pour the mixture into the prepared graham cracker crust.

4. Refrigerate for at least 4 hours before serving.

Prep Time: 15 minutes
Chill Time: 4 hours
Total Time: 4 hours, 15 minutes

7. Chocolate Chip Cookies

Ingredients:
2 1/2 cups of all-purpose flour
1 teaspoon of baking soda
1 teaspoon of salt
1 cup of butter, softened
3/4 cup of white sugar
3/4 cup of brown sugar
1 teaspoon of vanilla extract
2 eggs

2 cups of semi-sweet chocolate chips

Instructions:

1. Preheat the oven to 375 degrees Fahrenheit.

2. In a medium bowl, mix together the flour, baking soda, and salt. Set aside.

3. In a large bowl, cream together the butter, sugars, and vanilla extract.

4. Beat in the eggs one at a time.

5. Gradually add the flour mixture to the wet ingredients and mix until combined.

6. Stir in the chocolate chips.

7. Drop by rounded spoonfuls onto ungreased baking sheets.

8. Bake for 8-10 minutes or until golden brown.

Prep Time: 15 minutes
Cook Time: 8-10 minutes
Total Time: 23-25 minutes

8. Rice Pudding

Ingredients:
2 cups of cooked white rice
1/2 cup of raisins
4 cups of milk

1/2 cup of white sugar

1 teaspoon of ground cinnamon

1/2 teaspoon of ground nutmeg

1/4 teaspoon of salt

2 eggs, lightly beaten

Instructions:

1. Preheat the oven to 350 degrees Fahrenheit.

2. In a large bowl, combine the cooked rice, raisins, milk, sugar, cinnamon, nutmeg, and salt.

3. Stir in the eggs until well blended.

4. Pour the mixture into a 9x13 inch baking dish.

5. Bake in preheated oven for 30-40 minutes or until the top is golden brown.

Prep Time: 15 minutes
Cook Time: 30-40 minutes
Total Time: 45-55 minutes

9. Carrot Cake

Ingredients:
2 cups of all-purpose flour
2 teaspoons of baking powder
2 teaspoons of ground cinnamon
1/2 teaspoon of ground nutmeg
1/2 teaspoon of salt

3 eggs

1 cup of vegetable oil

2 cups of white sugar

3 teaspoons of vanilla extract

2 cups of grated carrots

Instructions:

1. Preheat the oven to 350 degrees Fahrenheit.

2. Grease and flour a 9x13 inch baking pan.

3. In a large bowl, combine the flour, baking powder, cinnamon, nutmeg, and salt.

4. In a separate bowl, beat together the eggs, oil, sugar, and vanilla extract.

5. Gradually add the dry ingredients to the wet ingredients and stir until well blended.

6. Fold in the grated carrots.

7. Pour the batter into the prepared pan and bake for 30-35 minutes or until a toothpick inserted into the center comes out clean.

Prep Time: 15 minutes
Cook Time: 30-35 minutes
Total Time: 45-50 minutes

10. Fruit Salad

Ingredients:
1 cup of blueberries

1 cup of strawberries, sliced

1 cup of raspberries

1 cup of blackberries

1/2 cup of white sugar

1/4 cup of orange juice

1/2 cup of chopped pecans

Instructions:

1. In a large bowl, combine the blueberries, strawberries, raspberries, and blackberries.

2. In a separate bowl, mix together the sugar and orange juice.

3. Pour the orange juice mixture over the fruit and stir until well combined.

4. Cover and refrigerate for at least 2 hours before serving.

5. Just before serving, stir in the chopped pecans.

Prep Time: 15 minutes
Chill Time: 2 hours
Total Time: 2 hours, 15 minutes

11. Cheesecake

Ingredients:
1 9-inch pre-made graham cracker crust
2 packages of cream cheese, softened
1 cup of white sugar
1 teaspoon of vanilla extract
2 eggs

3 tablespoons of all-purpose flour

1/2 cup of sour cream

Instructions:

1. Preheat the oven to 350 degrees Fahrenheit.

2. In a large bowl, beat together the cream cheese, sugar, and vanilla extract until smooth.

3. Beat in the eggs one at a time.

4. Gradually add the flour and mix until combined.

5. Stir in the sour cream.

6. Pour the mixture into the prepared graham cracker crust.

7. Bake in a preheated oven for 30-35 minutes or until the middle is almost set.

Prep Time: 15 minutes
Cook Time: 30-35 minutes
Total Time: 45-50 minutes

12. Strawberry Shortcake

Ingredients:
1 9-inch premade shortcake crust
1 quart of fresh strawberries, sliced
1/2 cup of white sugar
1 cup of heavy cream

Instructions:

1. Preheat the oven to 325 degrees Fahrenheit.

2. Place the shortcake crust in a 9-inch pie plate.

3. In a medium bowl, mix together the strawberries and sugar.

4. Pour the mixture into the shortcake crust.

5. Whip the heavy cream until stiff peaks form.

6. Spread the whipped cream over the top of the strawberry mixture.

7. Bake in a preheated oven for 20-25 minutes or until the top is golden brown.

Prep Time: 15 minutes
Cook Time: 20-25 minutes
Total Time: 35-40 minutes

13. Chocolate Fondu

Ingredients:
1 cup of semi-sweet chocolate chips
1/4 cup of heavy cream
1 teaspoon of vanilla extract
Assorted fresh fruit and pound cake, cut into cubes

Instructions:

1. In a medium saucepan, heat the chocolate chips and cream over low heat until melted and smooth.

2. Stir in the vanilla extract.

3. Transfer the mixture to a fondue pot or slow cooker.

4. Serve with fresh fruit and pound cake cubes for dipping.

Prep Time: 15 minutes
Cook Time: 10 minutes
Total Time: 25 minutes

14. Apple Crisp

Ingredients:

4 cups of sliced apples

1/2 cup of white sugar

1/2 cup of packed brown sugar

1/2 cup of all-purpose flour

1/2 teaspoon of ground cinnamon

1/4 teaspoon of ground nutmeg

1/4 cup of butter, melted

Instructions:

1. Preheat the oven to 375 degrees Fahrenheit.

2. Place the apples in a 9x13 inch baking dish.

3. In a medium bowl, mix together the sugars, flour, cinnamon, and nutmeg.

4. Stir in the melted butter until crumbly.

5. Sprinkle the mixture over the apples.

6. Bake in a preheated oven for 40-45 minutes or until the top is golden brown.

Prep Time: 15 minutes
Cook Time: 40-45 minutes
Total Time: 55-60 minutes

15. Baked Apples

Ingredients:
6 apples, peeled, cored, and halved

3 tablespoons of butter

3 tablespoons of white sugar

3 tablespoons of brown sugar

1/2 teaspoon of ground cinnamon

1/4 teaspoon of ground nutmeg

Instructions:

1. Preheat the oven to 350 degrees Fahrenheit.

2. Grease a 9x13 inch baking dish.

3. Place the apple halves in the prepared dish.

4. In a small bowl, mix together the butter, sugars, cinnamon, and nutmeg.

5. Spread the mixture over the apples.

6. Bake in a preheated oven for 30-35 minutes or until the apples are tender.

Prep Time: 15 minutes
Cook Time: 30-35 minutes
Total Time: 45-50 minutes

SMOOTHIES

1. Blueberry and Spinach Smoothie for Fertility

Introduction: This fertility smoothie is a delicious way to get your body ready for conception.

Blueberries are packed with antioxidants and vitamins that can help boost your fertility, while spinach is an excellent source of folic acid, which is vital for the health of both you and your baby.

Ingredients:

- ½ cup frozen blueberries

- 1 cup spinach

- ½ cup almond milk

- 1 tablespoon honey

- ½ banana

- 1 tablespoon chia seeds

Instructions:

1. Place all ingredients in a blender and blend until smooth.

2. Pour into a glass and enjoy!

Prep Time: 5 minutes

2. Avocado and Coconut Smoothie for Fertility

Introduction: Avocados are high in healthy fats and fiber, which can help boost fertility and regulate hormones.

Adding coconut to the mix provides a nutrient-rich boost to the smoothie, as well as a delicious tropical flavor.

Ingredients:

- ½ avocado
- ½ cup coconut milk
- ½ cup frozen pineapple
- 1 tablespoon honey
- ½ banana
- 1 teaspoon chia seeds

Instructions:

1. Place all ingredients in a blender and blend until smooth.

2. Pour into a glass and enjoy!

Prep Time: 5 minutes

3. Banana and Almond Butter Smoothie for Fertility

Introduction: This smoothie is a great way to get your fertility boost without overloading on sugar.

Bananas are high in potassium, a mineral that helps regulate hormones, and almond butter is packed with healthy fats that can help boost fertility.

Ingredients:
- 1 banana

- ½ cup almond milk

- 1 tablespoon almond butter

- 1 tablespoon honey

- ½ teaspoon cinnamon

- 1 teaspoon chia seeds

Instructions:

1. Place all ingredients in a blender and blend until smooth.

2. Pour into a glass and enjoy!

Prep Time: 5 minutes

4. Acai and Coconut Smoothie for Fertility
Introduction: This smoothie is a great way to get your fertility boost without overloading on sugar.

Acai berries are full of antioxidants, vitamins and minerals that can help boost fertility, while coconut adds a creamy texture and a delicious tropical flavor.

Ingredients:

- 1 packet frozen acai
- ½ cup coconut milk
- ½ cup frozen mango
- 1 tablespoon honey
- ½ banana
- 1 teaspoon chia seeds

Instructions:

1. Place all ingredients in a blender and blend until smooth.

2. Pour into a glass and enjoy!

Prep Time: 5 minutes

5. Strawberry and Mango Smoothie for Fertility

Introduction: This smoothie is a great way to get your fertility boost without overloading on sugar.

Strawberries are packed with antioxidants and vitamins that can help boost fertility, while mango adds a delicious tropical flavor.

Ingredients:
- ½ cup frozen strawberries
- ½ cup frozen mango
- ½ cup almond milk
- 1 tablespoon honey

- ½ banana

- 1 teaspoon chia seeds

Instructions:

1. Place all ingredients in a blender and blend until smooth.

2. Pour into a glass and enjoy!

Prep Time: 5 minutes

6. Peach and Almond Smoothie for Fertility

Introduction: Peaches are full of antioxidants and vitamins that can help boost fertility, while almond milk adds a creamy texture and a delicious nutty flavor.

Ingredients:

- ½ cup frozen peaches
- ½ cup almond milk
- 1 tablespoon almond butter
- 1 tablespoon honey
- ½ banana
- 1 teaspoon chia seeds

Instructions:

1. Place all ingredients in a blender and blend until smooth.

2. Pour into a glass and enjoy!

Prep Time: 5 minutes

7. Papaya and Coconut Smoothie for Fertility

Introduction: This smoothie is a great way to get your fertility boost without overloading on sugar.

Papaya is full of antioxidants, vitamins and minerals that can help boost fertility, while coconut adds a creamy texture and a delicious tropical flavor.

Ingredients:

- ½ cup frozen papaya
- ½ cup coconut milk
- 1 tablespoon honey
- ½ banana
- 1 teaspoon chia seeds

Instructions:

1. Place all ingredients in a blender and blend until smooth.

2. Pour into a glass and enjoy!

Prep Time: 5 minutes

8. Kiwi and Banana Smoothie for Fertility

Introduction: This smoothie is a great way to get your fertility boost without overloading on sugar.
Kiwi is full of antioxidants and vitamins that can help boost fertility, while banana adds a creamy texture and a delicious natural sweetness.

Ingredients:
- ½ cup frozen kiwi
- ½ cup almond milk
- 1 tablespoon honey

- ½ banana

- 1 teaspoon chia seeds

Instructions:

1. Place all ingredients in a blender and blend until smooth.

2. Pour into a glass and enjoy!

Prep Time: 5 minutes

9. Pineapple and Coconut Smoothie for Fertility

Introduction: This smoothie is a great way to get your fertility boost without overloading on sugar.

Pineapple is full of antioxidants, vitamins and minerals that can help boost fertility, while coconut adds a creamy texture and a delicious tropical flavor.

Ingredients:
- ½ cup frozen pineapple
- ½ cup coconut milk
- 1 tablespoon honey
- ½ banana
- 1 teaspoon chia seeds

Instructions:
1. Place all ingredients in a blender and blend until smooth.

2. Pour into a glass and enjoy!

Prep Time: 5 minutes

10. Mango and Carrot Smoothie for Fertility

Introduction: This smoothie is a great way to get your fertility boost without overloading on sugar.

Mangoes are full of antioxidants, vitamins and minerals that can help boost fertility, while carrots add a delicious natural sweetness and are full of beta carotene, which is essential for healthy conception.

Ingredients:
- ½ cup frozen mango
- ½ cup almond milk
- 1 tablespoon honey
- ½ cup grated carrot

- 1 teaspoon chia seeds

Instructions:

1. Place all ingredients in a blender and blend until smooth.

2. Pour into a glass and enjoy!

Prep Time: 5 minutes

11. Coconut and Papaya Smoothie for Fertility

Introduction: This smoothie is a great way to get your fertility boost without overloading on sugar.

Coconut adds a creamy texture and a delicious tropical flavor, while papaya is full of antioxidants, vitamins and minerals that can help boost fertility.

Ingredients:
- ½ cup coconut milk
- ½ cup frozen papaya
- 1 tablespoon honey
- ½ banana
- 1 teaspoon chia seeds

Instructions:
1. Place all ingredients in a blender and blend until smooth.

2. Pour into a glass and enjoy!

Prep Time: 5 minutes

12. Banana and Spinach Smoothie for Fertility

Introduction: This fertility smoothie is a delicious way to get your body ready for conception.

Bananas are high in potassium, a mineral that helps regulate hormones, while spinach is an excellent source of folic acid, which is vital for the health of both you and your baby.

Ingredients:
- 1 banana
- 1 cup spinach
- ½ cup almond milk
- 1 tablespoon honey
- ½ teaspoon cinnamon

- 1 teaspoon chia seeds

Instructions:

1. Place all ingredients in a blender and blend until smooth.

2. Pour into a glass and enjoy!

Prep Time: 5 minutes

13. Avocado and Banana Smoothie for Fertility

Introduction: This smoothie is a great way to get your fertility boost without overloading on sugar.

Avocados are high in healthy fats and fiber, which can help boost fertility and regulate hormones, while bananas add a creamy texture and a delicious natural sweetness.

Ingredients:

- ½ avocado

- ½ cup almond milk

- 1 tablespoon honey

- ½ banana

- 1 teaspoon chia seeds

Instructions:

1. Place all ingredients in a blender and blend until smooth.

2. Pour into a glass and enjoy!

Prep Time: 5 minutes

14. Acai and Banana Smoothie for Fertility

Introduction: This smoothie is a great way to get your fertility boost without overloading on sugar.

Acai berries are full of antioxidants, vitamins and minerals that can help boost fertility, while bananas add a creamy texture and a delicious natural sweetness.

Ingredients:
- 1 packet frozen acai
- ½ cup almond milk
- 1 tablespoon honey
- ½ banana
- 1 teaspoon chia seeds

Instructions:

1. Place all ingredients in a blender and blend until smooth.

2. Pour into a glass and enjoy!

Prep Time: 5 minutes

15. Peach and Banana Smoothie for Fertility

Introduction: This smoothie is a great way to get your fertility boost without overloading on sugar.

Peaches are full of antioxidants and vitamins that can help boost fertility, while bananas add a creamy texture and a delicious natural sweetness.

Ingredients:

- ½ cup frozen peaches
- ½ cup almond milk
- 1 tablespoon honey
- ½ banana
- 1 teaspoon chia seeds

Instructions:

1. Place all ingredients in a blender and blend until smooth.

2. Pour into a glass and enjoy!

Prep Time: 5 minutes

CONCLUSION

The Male Fertility Cookbook is an invaluable resource for any man who is trying to increase their fertility and improve their reproductive health.

A comprehensive list of fertility-boosting foods, recipes, and tips for healthy living, it is an excellent guide for any man who is looking to take control of their fertility and reproductive health, with its easy-to-follow instructions and easy-to-find ingredients, the Male Fertility Cookbook is the perfect way for any man to start on the path to improved fertility and better reproductive health.

Printed in Great Britain
by Amazon